The advantages of a vegetarian/vegan diet - a lie?

A critical reflection on vegetarian lifestyle

Autor:
Julian Ziegler

The adventages of avegetarian/ vegan diet - a lie?
A critical reflection on vegetarian lifestyle

A MaRindu UG (haftungsbeschänkt) published book

Published in Germany by MaRindu UG (haftungsbeschränkt).

www.marindu.com
E-mail: schnieder@marindu.de

Names: Julian Ziegler, author.
Titel: The adventages of avegetarian/ vegan diet - a lie?
ISBN: 9781798697214

Contents

Introduction

In this ebook, I'm going to alienate some friends here, but science is science: A massive study found that being vegan or vegetarian could benefit you in a lot of different ways, but it won't help you live longer.

Researchers tracked 243,096 men and women with an average age of 62. A six year follow up found that meat eaters and folks who followed a vegetarian diet or some version thereof (including vegetarianism "flirters") lived the same amount of time. Even after researchers adjusted for other factors like age, smoking, and diseases like type 2 diabetes, they found no evidence that forgoing meat could help you live longer.

What diet will help extend your life span?

Other studies came to the same conclusion. In fact, data from three cohort studies published earlier this year with around 200,000 American health workers found a vegetarian diet based on refined grains and other unhealthy foods could actually increase your risk for heart disease. Upon closer inspection, researchers found those eating a plant-based diet rich in fruits, vegetables, and healthy fats were less likely to get heart disease than people eating stuff like potatoes, refined grains, and sugar-loaded foods.

In other words, eating meat doesn't matter as much as eating quality food. Unfortunately, there's still a lot of confusion and contention about this: "It's not easy to know for sure what is the 'truth.' Vegan diet studies show they help with weight loss, reverse diabetes, and lower cholesterol.

Do vegans consume more vitamins and minerals?

Consider nutrients: Do plantbased eaters get more than meat eaters? One cohort study looked at 65,429 men and women between 20 and 97 with various dietary habits and backgrounds, including many non-meat eaters and meat eaters. Researchers compared overall nutrient intake and found vegetarians and vegans had the highest intakes of fiber, vitamin B1, folate, vitamin C, vitamin E, and magnesium. But they had the lowest intakes of retinol, vitamin B12, vitamin D, calcium, and zinc. Meat eaters got some of these nutrients, but they also consumed less fiber (bad) and more saturated fat (good or bad, depending on the source).

Another study found that in general, vegans and vegetarians ate more vegetables and legumes and less junk food than meat eaters. (They also took more supplements.) In other words, it might not be eliminating meat that creates longevity; it could be increased intake of nutrient-dense plant foods.

What role do lifestyle factors play here?

One study looked at the effects of lifestyle and food on chronic disease among vegetarians and vegans compared with meat eaters. Researchers found meat eaters had more chronic diseases like obesity, hypertension, and type 2 diabetes. Unfairly, higher saturated fat and cholesterol intake got the blame for this increased disease risk. But interestingly, meat eaters who practiced healthy lifestyle factors meaning they didn't smoke or drink excessive alcohol, they exercised regularly, and they consumed plenty of fruits and vegetables had results similar to those of vegetarians and vegans who also practiced healthy lifestyle factors.

From these and other studies, we can put together a more accurate picture on longevity. Research generally finds that vegetarians and vegans engage in healthier lifestyle practices than other groups, including meat eaters. (But that doesn't mean they all do.) From that perspective, one study found little difference in death rates between vegetarians and vegans and those who consume meat. Meat eaters who consumed more fruits and vegetables, didn't smoke, and exercised regularly had lower mortality rates than those who didn't maintain these and other lifestyle factors.

How can I live and eat in a way that promotes longevity?

Some studies show that consuming fruits and vegetables decreases stroke risk and lowers ischemic heart disease mortality, while increasing cardiovascular health regardless of whether or not you eat meat. Others show that lots of fruits and vegetables along with regular exercise influence cardiovascular health, blood pressure, triglycerides, and cholesterol levels. It can be overwhelming, but all this information isn't as confusing and contradictory as it seems when you focus on one idea: Eating more plant foods and living healthier, not necessarily entirely avoiding meat, seems the smarter path to longevity.

With that said, regardless of whether or not you eat meat, I've found these universal truths can bridge our differences and help us all become healthier:

1. Eat more plant foods.
Make about 75 percent of your plate plant foods like leafy and cruciferous vegetables. Regardless of whether you're vegan, vegetarian, or animal-based, make that other 25 percent protein- and healthy fat-rich foods.

2. Just eat real food, period.

Eat foods that are as close to nature as possible. If you couldn't hunt, pluck, gather, or otherwise find it in the wild, step far, far away. If your great grandmother wouldn't recommend it, put it back. (And if you eat animal foods, eat the highest quality foods you can afford!)

3. Stress less.

Humans weren't designed to hunch over a computer 10 hours a day or take the hectic train or bus for an hour each day. You can't eliminate stress, but you can minimize it. Step away, breathe deeply, do some yoga or meditation, and de-21st century.

4. Sleep more.

Whether you're the staunchest vegan or hard core carnivore, you're probably not getting enough quality sleep. Happy hour happens in your bed: Aim for eight hours nightly of deep, restorative sleep.

Historical / Anthropological / Philosophical aspects

The social sciences perspective: synthesis Veganism, as a lifestyle including and going beyond simple food choices, excludes all edible goods originating from animals.

Its underlying philosophical premise is based on an ethical principle that does not accord legitimacy or necessity to any form of animal exploitation. With roots dating back to Antiquity for vegetarianism, the current vegan eating style entered progressively in a successful era thanks to the best seller "Animal Liberation" published by the Australian philosopher and bioethician Peter Singer and the frequently mentioned "China Study"

Veganism has its roots in the vegetarianism of the 19th century. The term "vegan" itself was coined in Scotland in 1944 by Donald Watson et al.

Sociological or anthropological studies on veganism are rare, although this lifestyle attracts attention from the media and possibly a growing number of people, as can be observed by the frequency of the key word "vegan" in search machines e.g. Google

In Switzerland, the followers are mostly women and persons of a higher socioeconomic status than the average, according to data of the Federal Statistical Office

A more recent study suggests however, that more men than woman are vegan In this review, the French distinction between "végétalien" and "végane" will not be maintained. The first refers to an individual following a strict vegetarian diet that also excludes dairy products, eggs or honey.

The second defines a person following a vegan diet but also refraining from any form of exploitation of animals, not only for food, but also for clothing and other purposes, e.g. the consumption of any product derived from or tested on animals.

Veganism thus follows anti-speciesism principles of not discriminating against other animal species and respecting their different rights. According to this world view nothing justifies that animals are «naturally» available for human needs.

From a socio-anthropological perspective, veganism cannot be reduced to a homogeneous set of dietary and consumption practices defining a social group per se. The phenomenon should be seen as a lifestyle guided by an ethical deal and a personal fulfilment search whose meanings and motivations are variable and are part of a wider system of social representations and food trends that are linked with increasingly widespread values in Western societies. These representations and values are based on a reflexive and proactive attitude mainly in regard to exploitation and animal abuse, individual health and environmental sustainability.

Brief historical overview

Abstention of meat consumption punctuates Western history since Antiquity. The motivations of this opposition to an omnivore society are mainly based on the rejection of the ritual sacrifice of animals; this practice was seen as bloody and immoral by some philosophers such as Pythagoras, Theophrastos, Empedocle, Porphyros . The problem of suffering and of animal immolation as well as the belief in the metempsychosis (transmigration of the soul or reincarnation of the deceased in a living being, human or animal) divided also the first Christians .

At the end of the 18th century groups of Protestant dissidents first, followed by philanthropic movements, advocating vegetarianism appear in England. The utilitarian philosopher Jeremy Bentham asserted that the animal suffering, like the human suffering, was worthy of moral consideration, and he regarded cruelty to animals as analogous to racism.

The first vegetarian society was created in England in 1847 by members of the Bible Christian Church , and the International Vegetarian Union was founded in 1908. In Switzerland a vegetarian society was founded in 1880.

This spiritual and moral vegetarianism reached the United States during the 19th century where it was transformed into a hygienist movement. In the United States and in Europe, particularly in Switzerland and in Germany, an expansion of vegetarianism can be seen, particularly in health facilities applying the precepts of the „Lebensreform". Socio-symbolic dimensions of a vegan lifestyle choice

The three major motivations – compassion for the animals, quest for "pure" food and asceticism meatless diet advocated in Antiquity remain relevant (the first in particular) to understand the motivations and unconscious symbolic challenges of the contemporary veganism. Thus, in the heart of the "vegan culture" we find the conception of respect for animal life, which refers to the myth of paradise where people and animals used to live together peacefully, living exclusively on the fruits of a prodigal mother-earth. In this myth, violence inflicted on animals by men to dominate and feed on would ensue from a primordial sacrifice breaking the original harmony of the world and demanding, therefore, purifying rites (ritual slaughter) whose function is to "civilize" the act of killing. For anthropologists, this ritual sacrifice assumes a control function of so called "food murder", whose goal is to attest, by appealing to the sacred, symbolic discontinuity between humans and animals (including mammals) to legitimize and thus make edible the sacrificed being. However, the current antispecism stands on an ethical and moral vision that involves responsibility and even guilt in human domination and violent destruction of animals for consumption. The process that leads an individual to consume exclusively plant products reflects an ethical awareness and a critical choice (or even a duty) to break with properties, nutritional and symbolic, historically and culturally attributed to killed animal flesh. The meat diet is, in fact, ambivalently associated with force, with power, but also with impurity and sin. The ensuing a The Cathars, although piscivorous, are also an example. "food decision" is the result of a process of rationalization and incorporation by the individual, which, depending on its cultural frame of reference and its successive socializations, leads him to "choose" one or other diet and to define himself in relation to the "opposite" one.

Various studies point out that vegetarians are not a homogeneous entity. Their biographies, their motivations, their interests, their spirituality and their therapeutic approaches, nevertheless show some recurrences. It would be appropriate to apply this pluralistic approach to veganism too.

As shown by qualitative surveys collecting the stories of people having turned to vegetarianism , subjects explain their conversion - gradual or sudden – as having begun at key moments of their life cycle (adolescence, leaving home, birth of a child, separation, divorce...) or due to either serious or chronic health problems. The acute awareness of certain philosophical, ecological or political (North-South relations) themes also appears in the words of the respondents. Stories also refer to specific experiences that are often reliving memories of childhood or youth (like the "put to sleep" of a pet or a visit to a slaughterhouse). Especially older followers also describe forms of asceticism (fasting) and sexual abstinence. Even if one or the other pattern is predominant, motivations and practices often combine to result in a particular food order and a way of life (first meaning of the Greek term diaeta). The experience of the most convinced vegetarians tends to validate the thesis of a true "alternation", a conversion or transformation of a social identity resulting from the internalization of a different meaning system. Such experience is often described through evocation of emotionally strong moments, mention of resources and support from charismatic persons, length and density of learning, and comprehensive incorporation of experiences learned during internships and courses.

Environmental concerns also lead to a general preference for organically grown food .

In a German study with over 800 vegans the major motivations for choosing a vegan diet were objections to mass animal husbandry, environmental concerns and health issues.

In a USA study with both vegetarians and vegans (n=312), ethical reasons (animal rights, ethics, spiritual beliefs, environment and non-specified other ethical reasons) were more commonly (75%) given as a reason for becoming vegetarian / vegan. Health reasons (general health, weight loss, other health-related reasons) were mentioned by 18.5% of the participants, other minor reasons were taste, family/friends, upbringing, politics and saving money.

A recent qualitative study performed in Germany also concludes that ethical and political considerations are the main motivations for a vegan lifestyle.

Definitions and statistics

Vegetarian diets are plant-based diets, characterized by abstention from the consumtion of foods of animal origin, the extent of which can vary, but generally excludes consumption of animal flesh. Swiss food legislation has defined conditions required for the labelling of vegetarian foods.

a) "Vegetarian", or "ovo-lacto-vegetarian", whenever neither ingredients, nor processing aids, of animal origin are included, with the exception of milk, milk components, such as lactose, eggs, egg compo-nents and honey.
b) "Ovo-vegetarian", whenever neither ingredients, nor processing aids, of animal origin are included, with the exception of eggs, egg components, or honey.
c) "Lacto-vegetarian", whenever neither ingredients, nor processing aids, of animal origin are included, with the exception of milk, milk components and honey.
d) "Vegan", whenever no ingredients of animal origin are included.

These definitions are consistent with a large part of the reviewed literature where, however, veganism also excludes processing aids of animal origin. The scientific literature selected for this review included other definitions for vegetarian diets, mainly defined by the food groups of animal origin still included in the diet. This classification is not standardized, and most studies rely mainly on self-reporting or on general questions concerning intake of food items of animal origin, based on food frequency question-naires developed for the general, omnivorous population. In this review, focus will be on general vegan diets, extended to vegetarian diets only when the vegan data are insufficient.

Data on the prevalence of vegetarians and vegans in Switzerland are scarce and summarized below but suggest a range from 0.2% (menuCH data) to maximum 3% (Swissveg data) of the adult population following a vegan diet, and approximately 6% a vegetarian diet. A higher prevalence of vegan/veg-etarian woman compared to men is consistent with existing data.

Flexitarian: Occasional inclusion (less than once per week) of flesh foodstuff (meat, poultry and fish) and permits eating all other animal products (e.g. eggs, milk, honey).

General vegetarian diets: Whenever not specified, a vegetarian diet is often an ovo-lacto-vegetarian diet, as also defined in the Swiss Legislation.

Pescetarian: Includes seafood/fish, but not flesh of other animals (meat, poultry), and permits eating all other anima products (e.g. eggs, milk, honey). This diet is sometimes included in the semi-vegetarian group.

Pollo vegetarian: Poultry is the only animal flesh consumed, as well as dairy and egg products. This diet is sometimes included in the semi-vegetarian group.

Ovo-lacto-vegetarian: Excludes all types of flesh foodstuffs (meat, poultry, fish), but permits eating all other animal products (e.g. eggs, milk, honey).

Lacto-vegetarian: Excludes flesh foodstuffs and eggs but allows dairy products, honey.

Ovo-vegetarian: Excludes consumption of all animal products with the exception of eggs.

Vegan/ Vegetalian: Diet which excludes all animal products (both as ingredients and processing aids, the latter being an important aspect, not mentioned in the Swiss legislation).An exception is human mother's breast milk, given voluntarily. Veganism can also imply excluding all items of animal origin (e.g. made from wool, silk, leather materials). In French-speaking, areas a distinction is made between "végane" and "végétalisme". Other sub-categories of a vegan diet are:
-**Vitarian:** (raw vegan): Permits consumption of organic, raw and fresh foods only. Excludes coffee and tea.
-**Fruitarian:** Excludes flesh foodstuffs, animal products and vegetables, cereals permitted are only fruit, nuts, seeds, which can be gathered without damaging the plant
-**Sproutarian:** Eating foods in the form of sprouted plant seedlings, such as grains, vegetables, fruits.

Little is known about the typical duration of a vegan diet. The most recent study performed in Switzerland confirms that a majority of vegans (76%) have been following a vegan diet for less than five years, Schüpbach et al. report an average duration of 3.0 years (1.0-18.0). In a USA cross-sectional study with 312 vegetarians and vegans it was observed that participants choosing their diet for ethical reasons had been following the diet for a longer period (mean 9.97 years) than participants who mentioned health reasons (mean 5.9 years), this study is however based on self-reported data, and a selection/response bias is possible.

Even less is known about the prevalence of relapsed vegans. A cross-sectional survey performed in 2014 in the U.S.A. estimates a prevalence of 0.5% vegans, but of 1.1% former vegans. The data on the duration of the vegan diet are unclear, 34% of the former vegans followed this diet for less than three months. 37% of former vegans are however interested in re-adopting a vegan diet in future, often for health reasons. This survey suggests that some individuals will switch between omnivorous, vegetarian and vegan diets throughout their lifespan, and that even vegans cannot maintain an absolute diet purity. This type of eating pattern could alleviate some typical potential nutrient deficiencies discussed in the following chapters, in particular for vitamin B12, and health outcomes, but no specific studies were found on the topic.

Vegan diets from the nutrient perspective

Recent cross-sectional and cohort studies provide data on the diet of healthy adult vegetarian and vegans in Europe, these studies will be the main sources for assessing the potential nutrient-based risks and benefits linked with a vegan diet. In Switzerland, the dietary intake was assessed with a three-day weighed food record (analysed with the EBIS pro software) + questionnaire and measuring plasma concentrations of vitamins and minerals. In Denmark a four-day weighed food record was performed, using a 52-item FFQ (including vegan protein sources, such as tofu, meat alternatives) and the Danish FCDB40. In the United Kingdom the EPIC-Oxford cohort study used specific questionnaires, these results were updated in 2016. A further UK study was performed by analysing the data of the UK Biobank, based on 24-h dietary assessments. This study focused on protein intake and on protein sources. In Belgium dietary intake was assessed by FFQ and using a Belgian FCDB. In Finland a three-day food record was performed, combined with plasma, serum and urine analysis. In the French web-based NutriNet-Santé study dietary data were collected using 24-h reports and the daily nutrient intakes were calculated using a specific NutriNet FCDB, data were adjusted for sex, age and total energy intake.

Details for these studies are given in appendix II, due to methodological limitations these studies were clas-sified as being of evidence level C.

Macronutrient Intakes

Based on the dietary records rough estimates were made for the intake of macronutrients. This overview suggests that a vegan diet can cover the macronutrient recommendations (carbo-hydrates, fats, including low SFA, dietary fibre, total energy), as reported in all studies. The standard deviations are however wide, for the Swiss sample, the mean protein intake of 65g could corresponds to an adequate quantitative intake for healthy adults, but with a variability of +/- 21 g. Generally, these data indicate that some participants are not covering their protein needs. The published data do not however pro-vide specifics on the participants with the lower protein intake, e.g. gender, age, body weight, PAL. None of the studies specifically described a protein deficiency. The small number of participants and a possible se-lection bias (intrinsic motivation of participants to participate, "healthy volunteer effect") must however be considered.

Even in a well-balanced omnivore diet, about 30-40% of the protein intake is provided by food of plant origin. This percentage increases when protein-rich vegetable products (e.g. pulses, soybean-based products) are included: An adequate intake of these food items theoretically covers protein needs. The essential amino acid needs could also be covered, by eating a variety of protein–rich foods during the day. In the EPIC-Oxford study qualitative aspects of the protein intake were assessed with a cross-sectional analysis. Vegans (n=98) covered 2.8% of their energy intake with protein from soya products and 9.6% with protein from non-soya plant products, the intake profiles for amino acids was significantly lower than those of all other diet groups, in particular for essential amino acids.

Both vegetarian and vegan diets had a lower intake of non-essential amino acids, com-pared to omnivores. Plasma analysis however, showed that only few amino acids (lysine, methionine and tryptophan) were significantly lower in vegans. These studies all show that attention is needed to cover both qualitative and quantitative (amino acid) needs. Furthermore, other aspects, such as the possibly lower di-gestibility and skeletal muscle anabolic response to plant proteins, were not taken into account.

These results show that for the assessment of the nutritional status more accurate data are needed, e.g. there is a suspicion of under-reporting in the UK data, the data should be stratified at least by sex. The data do not take into consideration finer details, such as the impact of the underlying motivation for following a vegan diet, which could have an impact on the eating pattern. The most recent Swiss study shows that most vegans are motivated by ethical and environmental concerns, only 35% follow this diet for health reasons.

As recognized by Radnitz et al. with an international online survey (n=246 participants) health-based or ethically-based vegan choices can influence the eating patterns, with the first (health motivated vegans) more frequently associated with healthier food choices (more fruit and fewer sweets), whereas ethically driven vegans reported a higher likelihood of taking supplements, soy-based products, and high-polyphenol bever-ages. Dyett et al also report different lifestyle and dietary behaviours among the 100 USA study participants, depending on the underlying reason for their vegan choice.

When comparing the Swiss vegan/vegetarian data with the average data collected during the Swiss survey menuCH51 the energy, fat and carbohydrate intakes are comparable to the general study, with however a lower protein intake and a higher dietary fibre intake. Further research is necessary in evaluating if differences in eating patterns, depending on the motivation, could impact the macronutrient intakes.

Positive nutrient aspects of a vegan diet

In general all diet forms providing a high intake of fruit and vegetables have a positive effect on health, as confirmed most recently by Aune et al. The above-mentioned studies do not however report the estimated intake of different food items, which would be of great interest, because it is generally assumed that a vegan diet is rich in fruit and vegetables. This assumption was one of the salient basis of the former FCN report. Some fruit and vegetable intake data have been published and are summarized in table below. Vegan diets include more fruit and vegetables than other diets, the average values show that general recommendations of 2 portions of fruits (200-240 g) and 3 portions of vegetables (300-360 g) are fulfilled. These data show however, that fruit and vegetable intakes vary among the different studies, furthermore, the standard varia-tions, when reported, indicate a wide variability in intakes in the individual studies. Based on the data it is not evident to conclude that a vegan diet is per default rich in fruits and vegetables. Therefore, not all vegans can unquestionably benefit from the advantages of a plant-based diet with a high fruit and vegetable intake (i.e. with more than 4-5 portions of vegetables and fruits per day).

A balanced vegan diet can cover macronutrient needs, as seen above. In the Belgian study food intake data were evaluated with a Healthy Eating Index and the vegan diets were shown to have the highest scoring with this index, compared to the omnivores in the study group. A high intake of foods of plant origin (fruit, vegetables, cereals, pulses and nuts), covers the needs of many micronutrients typically found in these food groups. Compared to ovo-lacto-vegetarians and omnivores, vegans have a higher intake resp. status for several nutrients: magnesium, vitamins C, B1, B6, folic acid, as recorded and measured in the Swiss study by Schüpbach et al. It can be expected that a vegan diet also provides a wide array of phytochemicals (e.g. carotenoids, phenolics), with potential health benefits.

As described by Platel et al. for example the use of spices, onions and garlic as well as acidic fruits in the diet enhances the bioavailability of trace elements (e.g. iron) from plant foods. This may contribute to a sufficient supply with trace elements from sources with rather poor bioavailability and could counter the negative effect of phytic acid.

Micronutrient deficiency risks of a vegan diet

When assessing the micronutrient intake of vegans, care should be taken into recording accurately any supplement intake. A German qualitative study (5 focus groups in different locations with a total of 42 vegan participants) confirms that a minority of vegans do not see the necessity of a supplementation, believing that a well-balanced vegan diet provides all necessary nutrients. Supplements are however recommended by vegan societies, e.g. the Swiss Vegan Society, in particular for vitamin B1216. European studies show that not all vegans follow this recommendation.

Estimates in the micronutrient intake are often based on food intake, and do not take into account variations in the bioavailability and absorption rates of each micronutrient. Blood and/or urine samplings are therefore more appropriate as biomarkers for the effective micronutrient status.

Schüpbach et al. show that all diet groups show low intakes / status for some micronutrients. Although the average micronutrient intakes seem to be in the normal reference ranges, with the exception of iron, resp. its biomarker plasma ferritin, the percentage of vegan participants below the cut-offs for deficiencies is crit-ical for selected nutrients (Zn, I, B2, B6). This will be discussed in more detail below, together with other potentially critical micronutrients, discussed in alphabetical order.

Calcium

In omnivore resp. lactovegetarian diets, milk and dairy products often represent a major dietary source for calcium. Well-planned vegan diets can include sufficient calcium-rich sources, such as green vegetables, nuts and pulses, sme mineral waters, and/or calcium-enriched products. Most studies compared actual intake data to the recommended intake of 800 mg. The DACH reference value for adults was increased to 1000 mg Ca suggesting that for many vegans a dietary adjustment / supplementation is necessary.

Some typical examples of naturally calcium-rich food items would be: broccoli (93 mg/100 g), sesame seed (940 mg/100 g), generic mineral water (up to 50 mg/100 ml), pulses, e.g. lentils (57 mg/100 g dry product), dry soybeans (200 mg/100 g). The Schüpbach et al. study shows that 54% of the vegan participants con-sumed less than 800 mg Ca/day, whereas only 17% of the vegetarians and 28% of the omnivores did not reach this intake target. The mean Ca intake for the vegan participants was however of 817 mg/day (+/- 285), thus demonstrating that some vegan diets provide an adequate calcium intake. Similar results are reported in the Belgian study, with a mean intake of 730 mg Ca/day; the Finland study reports a mean of 1'004 mg Ca/day for the vegan population, which is only slightly lower compared to the matched non-vegetarian group, with 1'117 mg Ca.

The EPIC cohort was investigated by different groups (for detail refer to appendix II). An adjusted mean calculated intake of 848 mg Ca in the vegan group, with 17.1% of female participants, and 13.5% of male participants not achieving the estimated average requirements. The investigation on diet and fracture risk. The baseline characteristics showed a mean calcium intake for male: meat-eaters 1'062 mg (+/-325), fish-eaters 1'086 mg (+/-355), vegetarians 1'085 mg (+/-1'085) and vegans 603 mg (+/-232). For women the figures were only slightly lower: meat-eaters 995 mg (+/-303), fish-eaters 1'029 mg (+/-337), vegetarians 1'018 mg (+/-357) and vegans 586 mg (+/-226). The pooled intake of men and women was below 525 mg for 44.5% of the subjects, possibly associated with an increased fracture risk.

A second concern is the bioavailability of these calcium sources, considering that vegetables and pulses also contain variable quantities of calcium-binding organic acids (such as phytic and oxalic acid). As there is a lack of food composition data, it could be helpful to plan a calcium-rich diet, preferring food items with lower phytic or oxalic acid contents.

The importance of an adequate calcium intake in children is discussed , A long-term calcium deficiency could affect bone health; however, a vegan diet could possibly also include bone-protecting components. The impact of a vegan diet on bone health is discussed.

Iodine

Iodine is frequently mentioned as a critical element in vegan diets, e.g. by the German Society of Nutrition. The situation in Switzerland is different, as without the fortification of salt, iodine deficiency would be en-demic for the whole population. The fortification of salt has helped fulfilling the population target intake levels (150 g / d). The iodine status is regularly monitored. Results of iodine monitoring campaigns up to 2009 led to a mandatory increase of the iodine content of iodized salt from 20 to 25 mg/kg in January 2014.

Although iodized salt is the main source of iodine in Swiss diets, its use is not mandatory; the use of uniodized salts (both in industrial foods and/or household salt) is frequent. The recent menuCH survey reports that 69% of the participants use iodized salt in their household, showing a reduction from the 80% recorded in the last iodine monitoring. Chappuis et al. investigated the use of iodized salt in the general Swiss adult population and observed that over a third of the survey participants do not regularly use iodized salt.

Specific data on the use of iodized salt for vegans who cannot rely on sea fish or cow's milk for their iodine supply. Including seaweed in the diet could lead to higher iodine intake; the frequency in use of these algal sources is unknown. No further data was found on the calculated iodine intake in the vegan subjects in the Swiss studies.

Urine iodine values were calculated in the recent study from Schüpbach et al. The median concentrations range from 83 µg/l in omnivores to 75 µg/l in vegetarians (not a significant difference) to a significantly lower 56 µg/l in vegans. In all three dietary groups a majority ($\geq$ 65%) does not reach the cut-off value of 100 µg/l currently recommended by the WHO. Similar trends were observed in the plasma data, with 78.8% of vegans below the cut-off for deficiency.

The iodine status for a larger sample of the Swiss population (n=1481) was assessed during the Swiss survey by Haldimann et al. on salt intake 2010-2012. The median urinary concentration was of overall 75.7 µg/l, thus in a similar range as the results for omnivores (83 µg/l) in the Schüpbach et al. study. The significant difference between women (62.5 µg/l) and men (90.6 µg/l), in the Haldimann et al study, suggests that the vegan data should be analysed for gender differences, in order to assess the potentially higher prevalence of an iodine deficiency in vegan women.

These results show that although iodine supplementation is necessary for the Swiss population, vegans are at higher risk, which could lead to a reduced formation of active thyroid hormones. This however depends not only on a sufficient intake of iodine.

Iron

Iron is often mentioned as critical mineral for vegetarians and vegans e.g.9,68,69, recommended intakes vary, depending on different institutions, e.g. DACH reference values 10 mg (for males) / 10-15 mg (and for post-resp. premenopausal women).

In a healthy Swiss population the calculated average daily intake of iron was highest in vegans (median 22.9 mg, 12.8-43.0), followed by vegetarians (median 14.7 mg, 7.7-44.3) and omnivores (median 11.8 mg, 7.2-43.3). Iron can be found in plants and in food of animal sources in different forms. Plants contain mainly Fe3+, a non-heme iron, with limited bioavailability, unless consumed concomitantly with ascorbic acid-con-taining food, which reduces this iron to Fe2+. Food of plant origin also contains iron in form of phyto-ferritin: e.g. 40-90% of iron in pulses is in this form. Investigations show that this iron form possibly has a good bioavailability, the hypothesis being that it can be taken up by endocytosis, as based on tests with cultured cells.

Schüpbach et al further analysed plasma levels for haemoglobin and ferritin. All three groups held the same haemoglobin status (145 -147 g/l +/- 11-14), but different plasma ferritin (PF) levels. Omnivores had the highest median levels (58 g/l), vegetarians the lowest (32 g/l), vegans lay between the two other groups (40 g/l), the data collected from the vegan group were however not statistically different from that of omnivores, resp. vegetarians. The authors claim that for all three groups the plasma ferritin levels lay well within the normal range of 15-300 g ferritin/ l, without clinical symptoms. The Swiss Medical Board however rec-ommends a cut-off value of 50 g/l, the Swiss data of the Schüpbach study should be re-analysed in regard to this reference value, in order to have a better estimate of the percentage of participants below this cut-off value.

In the mentioned Belgian study, the calculated intake of iron is the highest in vegans, followed by vegetari-ans, and with the lowest calculated intake in the omnivore group. The calculations were based on the FFQ and a Belgian FCDB. These results do not take into account the bioavailability of the different forms of iron (Fe3+/Fe2+/ferritin and /or heme iron), and no blood sampling was performed44. The Finnish study also shows a non-significant higher intake of iron in the vegan group (21 mg +/-9 vs. 15 mg +/-7 in the non-vegetarian), the median ferritin levels in serum were however lower (26 µg/l vs 72 µg/l), both in the reference range, even when stratified (male/female).

Long-chain polyunsaturated n-3 fatty acids

Very-long chain polyunsaturated n-3 fatty acids (C20-C22) such as eicosapentaenoic acid (EPA, C20:5) and docosahexaenoic acid (DHA, C22:6) are important constituents of cell membrane lipids; in particular, DHA is enriched in brain lipids and in the photosensitive rod inner membranes of the eye. EPA is a precursor for several series of bioactive molecules, participating among other functions in blood clotting, inflammatory processes, secretory activities. Very low DHA levels are associated with depression and neurological dis-turbances. Specific aspects of the essentiality of EPA and DHA during neurological development of the fetus and after birth are discussed.

Omnivores, pescetarians and (ovo-)lactovegetarians have a supply of EPA and DHA in their diet; e.g. fatty fish is a good nutritional source for DHA.

In most studies, intake estimates are aggregated for all polyunsaturated fatty acids. These studies show slightly higher PUFA intakes for vegan than omnivores (values, adjusted for age and sex, vary among the studies: vegans 21-26 g PUFA, omnivores 15-22 g PUFA). The specific intake of n-3 fatty acids is not calculated in these studies. One Australian study shows that vegans have an intake of 84 mg n-3 fatty acids / day, whereas omnivores had an intake of 216 mg. Sanders reviews older literature and mentions intakes of ALA 2.2 g/day for vegans and 1.3 g for omnivores.

Vegans show very low levels of DHA in their circulating lipids, but not lower than omnivores who have a limited intake of DHA+EPA. Some authors prefer measuring the erythrocyte fatty acid composition (e.g. an Omega 3-Index) as an indicator for long-term intake of long-chain PUFAs60 as a potential biomarker for CHD risk, this approach has yet to be validated.

Low dose EPA+DHA-supplements can markedly elevate the blood DHA and EPA levels. A supplementa-tion is of particular important in life stages with higher requirements, such as pregnancy, lactation, or child-hood.

As some algae build directly DHA, vegan DHA supplements are available. Vegetarians and vegans should also prefer ALA-rich oils instead of oils rich in linoleic acid. Good ALA sources are rapeseed (canola) oil and walnuts; other ALA-rich oils, such as flaxseed, walnut and chia oils are very prone to oxidation reactions.

Humans are able to elongate and desaturate α-linolenic acid (ALA, C18:3), an essential n-3-precursor fatty acid, to EPA and, to a minor extent, to DHA. Linoleic acid (n-6) competes with ALA for the enzyme binding sites. Since normally the amount of linoleic acid in the diet exceeds by far the amount of ALA, the formation of EPA and DHA stays very modest in comparison to the formation of arachidonic acid, the n-6 compound corresponding to EPA. The endogenous conversion of ALA to EPA and DHA is limited, but evidence suggests that it might be sufficient to lead to stable DHA and EPA levels in vegans over many years. This process is dependent on metabolic genetics, age (decline with age), sex (less conversion in young males), health status (chronic disease, smoking), and dietary composition.

Selenium

The DACH recommended intake for selenium is of 70 (m)/60 (f) g/d. It is an essential trace element with functions as seleno-cystein in the active centre of several important enzymes. The antioxidant capacity depends amongst others on Se-containing peroxidases and thioreductases. The formation of functional thyroid hormone T3 depends on deiodinases, which are also selenoproteins. Today many human seleno-proteins have been identified, but their functions are still not fully elucidated. Deficiencies in selenium supply induce health problems concerning the muscles, the heart and the immune system85. The existing data on low selenium status and colorectal cancer risks in vegetarians are non-conclusive.

European soils contain less selenium than e.g. North American soils, as previously reported by Zimmerli. More recent research warns that climatic changes could exacerbate the problem of selenium depletion. Imported cereals therefore often cover selenium needs. Choosing regionally and organically grown cereals (e.g. without a specific selenium-containing fertilizer) could lead to decreased selenium intake, even for omnivores.

There are already some concerns about a generalized suboptimal selenium status in Europe. Data are missing on calculated dietary intakes, however the selenium status in blood is regularly monitored in Swit-zerland, with the most recent monitoring concluding that with an overall mean serum concentration of 98 µg/l (n=1'847), the selenium status of the healthy adults can be assessed as adequate". Recent analysis has confirmed that the intake of selenium corresponds directly to the plasma levels. Data on the selenium plasma levels in vegetarian or vegan population groups in Switzerland are scarce. The most recent study by Schüpbach et al. found no relevant differences in serum selenium concentrations between omni-vores, vegetarians and vegans, with values between 90 and 94 µg/l, the vegan had the greatest variability, 90 µg/l +/-21.9, suggesting that some vegans are at the lowest end of the recommended range of 70-150 µg/l.

Vitamin B12

The DACH recommended intake for vitamin B12 is 3 g/d (for the general adult population). Vitamin B12 is synthesized by some bacteria and is bio-accumulated along the food chain, supplementation with either cobalt (ruminants) or vitamin B12 (non-ruminants) is common in animal husbandry. In an omnivore diet meat from ruminants, is a good source for this vitamin (e.g. 2 µg/100 g beef filet). Minor sources of vitamin B12 are fermented products, in particular dairy products (e.g. 2 µg/100 g Gruyère-type cheese, 0.5 µg/100g yoghurt); all data from the Swiss FCDB; a detailed overview of vitamin B12 content of different meat types is provided by Gille & Schmid. Fermented plant-based food (e.g. sauerkraut, tempeh) contain traces of vitamin B12; precise data for products on the Swiss market are however missing.

Other possible vegan sources of vitamin B12 exist, e.g. Chlorella algae containing 3.9 -11.4 ng cyano-cobalamin/30 g algae, these quantities are however extremely low. Purple laver (nori) and some mushrooms have also been mentioned as possible active vitamin B12 sources. These are not necessarily frequent items in Western diets; for more data, they should be included in vegan-appropriate FFQs and reliable reference composition data are needed.

The uptake of this vitamin in the human body is mainly possible with the assistance of transport proteins, salivary R proteins, followed by the intrinsic factor (IF) produced by the stomach mucosa. Active absorption occurs in the distal part (ileum) of the gut, and is probably limited to 1.5-2 µg/meal; furthermore, the ab-sorption capacity decreases with age. The main cause for decreased absorption is an impaired secretion of gastric acid and IF due to mucosal inflammation, e.g. as a consequence of a long-term intake of proton-pump inhibitors. Mucosal inflammation becomes more prevalent with age (atrophic gastritis), leading to a decreased release of cobalamins from the proteins due to impaired protein denaturation and therefore de-creased absorption. These aspects must be considered when assessing vitamin B12 intake as the calculated intake, based on dietary assessments and FCDM alone could overestimate the effectively absorbed amount. Reports results of the studies comparing the calculated dietary intake (excluding supplements) with an estimated average requirement (EAR) of 2 µg/day showing that this requirement is not reached by vegans. This EAR is below the D-A-CH reference value of 3 µg for healthy adults, as well as below the adequate intake (AI) of 4 µg proposed by the European Food Safety Authority.

Serum B12 is traditionally used as a biomarker for bioavailable B12 (from dietary intake and / or depletion of the hepatic store) and has been used to assess the vitamin status in vegetarians. A review of the literature up to 2012 shows that vegans are at higher risk of a vitamin B12 deficiency. More than 50% of the participants had serum values below the cut-off range of 120-180 pmol/l. The Finnish study reports high median serum values of 328 pmol/l for vegans, 508 pmol/l for non-vegetarians. The Swiss study is more difficult to eval-uate, 43% of the participants were taking supplements up to 14 days before the study and had serum values of 342 pmol/l, those without supplementation had a high median value of 274 pmol/l. Only 7.5% of the vegan participants showed a deficiency. The authors conclude that the B12 status thus measured does not reflect the possibility of depletion of the body storages. Lacking awareness of the slow depletion of vitamin B12 stores could also be a factor leading to the denial of the necessity of a supplementation; indeed, high serum B12 values in the initial vegan phase can be erroneously used as proof that a supplementation is not neces-sary.

Serum B12 is therefore not the only biomarker, which should be taken into consideration.

Other markers recommended by these authors, with holo-transcobalamin II being the most frequently recommended analysis. A higher folic acid intake (typical of a vegan diet) could mask vitamin B12 deficiency symptoms if only a macrocytic anemia is being searched for.

Vitamin B12 supplementation is highly recommended for all vegans, this recommendation is not followed by all. Anecdotal evidence points to a certain resistance, so called "chemophobia" to supplements produced by biotechnological methods. Whilst this does not seem to be the case in the majority of vegans, this is often true for the smaller sub-population of vegans, e.g. raw vegans, and Rasta-farian vegans (who eschew both preservatives and vitamin supplementation).

Zinc

The DACH recommended intake for zinc is 10 mg/d (males) and 7 mg/d (females). This element is frequently mentioned as a critical element for vegetarians and vegans. It is a very important trace element with multiple functions in the human body. It is needed as cofactor in several hundred enzymes and proteins, participates in transcription and translation processes, thus influences growth, the secretion of hormones, the formation and growth of bones and stimulates responses of the immune system. Zinc is found mainly in protein rich food, both of animal and plant origin. As some vegans may consume less protein than rec-ommended , their zinc intake could be lower; furthermore, the bioavailability of zinc has to be taken into account. A comparative meta-analysis concluded that zinc intake and serum zinc levels are lower in populations following vegetarian diets, stressing that the variability of vegetarian diets made com-parisons difficult. In further analyses, the vegan groups had the lowest zinc serum values and zinc in-takes. The adjusted calculated mean zinc intake in the EPIC study was also significantly lower in the vegan group (8.7 mg) than in the vegetarian group (10.3 mg) and in the meat-eating group (10.5 mg). In an Australian study with young woman (n=308), micronutrient intake was assessed by FFQ, using the Aus-tralian FCDB. Participants were classified according to their avoidance of specific animal-derived products, "non-avoiders" could be considered omnivores (with a zinc intake of 15 mg, SD of 5), "avoiders of all" could be considered vegans (with a significantly lower zinc intake of 12 mg, SD 3). The higher Australian values lead to the question whether Australian products are naturally higher in zinc, making comparisons difficult.

In the Swiss study, the average daily intake of zinc was comparable in all three-diet groups and well above the estimated average requirement (EAR) for this element. However, the blood levels differed significantly for each group with the highest level in omnivores, followed by the vegetarians and the lowest level in vegans. Consequently, 47% of the vegan subjects had blood levels below the cut-off values (74 g / dl for men, 70 g / dl for women). In the vegetarian group this was the case for 19% and in the omnivorous group for 11% of the participants, the difference between the vegetarian and omnivorous groups is not significant.

These results show that calculated zinc intakes, based on FFQ and generic zinc contents of food items do not reflect the bioavailability of zinc and confirm the risk of zinc deficiency in vegan diets. This is of concern for all age groups, in particular however in infancy, childhood, pregnancy and breastfeeding, where physio-logical demands are higher.

Saunders et al point out that a major factor affecting zinc bioavailability is phytic acid, and suggests pro-cessing food in order to decrease the phytic acid / phytate content (e.g. enzymatically) or zinc supplemen-tation105. A molar ratio phytic acid: zinc of > 15 is considered to decrease the bioavailability of dietary zinc.

Unfortunately neither the Swiss FCDB, nor the frequently cited German FCDB (Bundes Lebensmittelschlüssel, BLS) lists phytic acid content. Some data were found in the "Souci" database and are summarized below. If this data is correct, in many food items of plant origin the phytic acid: zinc ratio is > 15.

No further data were found for a wider selection of pulses, soy products and other typical plant-based protein sources.

Zinc deficiency is also widespread in low-income countries, a Swiss study shows that specific treatment of cereals, e.g. the enzymatic dephytinization of oats, leads to an increase of the bioavailability of zinc. The same authors demonstrate the benefits of a zinc fortification.

Further risks of vegan diets

Dietary shifts towards more food of plant origin could lead to shifts in the exposition of specific food-associ-ated contaminants. The exposition to methylmercury, dioxins, polychlorinated biphenyls etc., typically accu-mulated in fatty foods of animal origin, is expected to be lower in a vegan or vegetarian diet; whereas a higher exposition is expected to typical contaminants in food of plant origin, e.g. arsenic in rice products, specific pesticides, cadmium. For arsenic, no Swiss data were found related to dietary patterns, but Japanese data indicate that rice based products, which would typically be part of a vegan diet, could be contaminated with arsenic. Monitoring of dietary arsenic in Switzerland has now become necessary, due to the introduction of cutoff values for arsenic with the Swiss food legislation reform in 2017.

Vegan diet could lead to an increased exposure to specific pesticide residues in France (triallate, and organophosphates (OPs) such as chlorpyrifos-methyl and diazinon).

Berman et al measured urinary levels of pesticides in individuals, stratified by different dietary patterns in the vegetarian and vegan Jewish Amirim community in Northern Israel. Focus was made on OPs and carbamates, which are widely used in the Israeli agriculture. Dietary exposure was measured by the ex-creted metabolites of these pesticides. Higher values were found, when comparing the Amirim sample of to those of a wider Israeli Jewish sample. These values were found to be associated with the higher intake of fruit (25% of the caloric intake, compared to 6% for the reference group) and vegetables (31% of the caloric intake, compared to 10% for the reference group). When organic produce was preferred, lower values for excreted OP metabolites were observed. This study has some limitations for its use in comparison with other data, in particular for the data on fruit and vegetable consumption, e.g. the classification of food items.

The data from France and Israel show that patterns in pesticide residues depend on the dietary patterns. OP-levels could be monitored in connection with a vegan/vegetarian diet. Furthermore, the extent of consumption of organic produce could also be relevant, and could be assessed in case of a monitoring.

Life cycle aspects of Vegan diets

Pregnancy and breastfeeding

The impact of a vegan diet during pregnancy and in the preconceptional phase is still a little-researched topic, specific case-reports, cross-sectional data, and prospective longitudinal data are still lacking. Older data are summarized by Cofnas, showing that nutrient deficiencies during pregnancy could be potentially harmful for the foetus.

Therefore, individual medical and dietetic counselling is highly recommended for women desiring to follow a strict vegan diet during pregnancy and lactatio. The reasons and motivation for a plant based diet should be evaluated; as seen in the previous chapter. Piccoli et al. found in their narrative review that only iron and vitamin B12 could be critical in some vegan or vegetarian diets, particularly when the increased needs for iron and vitamin B12 supplementation are not taken into account.

Pistollato et al. reviewed the existing literature and summarize further possible issues related to maternal plant-based dietary patterns. Main issues these authors are the lower intake of n-3 PUFAs (with possible negative outcomes for children), lower B12 intake, lower mineral intake (iron, zinc, iodine and calcium), as well as vitamin D deficiencies.

The source of iron in a vegan diet can influence absorption rates, leading to variable hemoglobin and ferritin levels for vegans. An iron deficiency can lead to anemia. In Switzerland, it is recom-mended to test hemoglobin and ferritin at the beginning of pregnancy in all women before treating them for anemia or iron deficiency, independently of their dietary choices. Vitamin B12 should be tested for women following a vegetarian or vegan diet: starting with vitamin B12 in serum, followed, in case of deficiency (or near-deficiency), by HoloTCII and MMA testing, and supplemented according to results. Supplementation should be continued into the lactation phase.

A vegan diet can lead to a higher intake of phytoestrogens (contained e.g. in soy-based products, linseed), with conflicting data on the possible risk of hypospadias, i.e. abnormal location of the urinal opening in the penis, further studies are needed to confirm this hypothesis.

Independently of the diet form, vitamin D supplementation (600 IU/day) is recommended for all pregnant women.

Pregnant and lactating vegetarian women who avoid seafood and algae and live in an area where the soil is deficient in iodine may have insufficient iodine intake to meet the needs of the fetus and the breastfed baby, with hypothyroidism as a consequence. The FCN report on iodine stated that a mild to moderate iodine deficiency is prevalent among pregnant and lactating women in Switzerland, because iodine needs increase to a minimum of 250 µg, this corresponds to the "DACH reference values of 230µg (pregnancy) to 260 µg (while breastfeeding) . Consequently, the FCN recommended all pregnant and lactating women to use iodized table salts available in Switzerland. The 2016 iodine survey for Switzerland shows a decrease in the urinary iodine concentration in pregnant women from 162 µg/l in 2009 to 140 µg/l in 2015 despite an increase in iodine concentration in salt in 2014. Therefore, a separate supplementation, besides iodized table salt, with 150 µg should be considered. Otherwise, deficiencies are likely, with important conse-quences for the development of children.

The zinc status during pregnancy has been object of a review and meta-analysis, comparing vegetarian to non-vegetarian (omnivore) women, but not specifically vegan women. Not only intake estimates, but also several biomarkers were used (serum/plasma, urine, hair samples). Most studies showed that the zinc sta-tus was lower in the vegetarian groups than in the non-vegetarian (omnivore) groups; both were however below the recommended levels.

A vegan diet is not recommended during pregnancy according to general dietary recommendations by one of the standard references in the German-speaking area, Koletzko et al. However, if a vegan diet is strongly desired by the pregnant woman, specific blood analysis, based on an individual dietary assess-ment, followed by medical and nutritional counselling and supplementation are necessary, taking into ac-count the generally recognized target nutrient intakes for pregnancy and lactaction.

Progress in the general physiological understanding of nutrient needs during pregnancy (e.g. iodine refer-ence values) has to be taken into account and included in dietary guidelines for pregnancy.

Infants / children

Little is known about the prevalence of infants and children fed on a vegan diet in Switzerland. In a large German nutritional survey (KiGGS-Study) only 1.7% of boys and 3.2% of girls older than 3 years reported being on a vegetarian diet, no information is available about children on an exclusively vegan diet.

When choosing a particular diet for a child, caregivers should be aware that the consumed food will form the basis for the rapidly developing biological organism.

This development is not only reflected in growth and weight gaining but on a much smaller scale in synap-togenesis within the central nervous system, specific gene activation or silencing, immune competence, allergy predisposition, even emotions and cognitive potential are influenced by the choice for and the quality of the food consumed. The type of early nutrition has furthermore an influence on feeding preferences when becoming an adult. When parents / caregivers decide on a vegan diet for their young children, they depart from well-established feeding patterns and assume thereby the whole responsibility of providing an adequate nutrition for their children. We do not know of any study conducted to investigate possible long-term health benefit of a well-planned vegan diet started in pediatric age. Due to the limited data on the impact of vegetarian diets in childhood, it is therefore difficult to draw conclusions on health benefits or risks of these diets.

More is known about particular aspects within a vegan diet such as energy supply, protein composition, and supply of long chain fatty acids, iron, zinc, vitamin D, iodine, calcium and vitamin B12. In the following sub-chapters, emphasis will be laid on the expected effects if the age dependent mini-mum requirements for a child cannot be met. The knowledge about these potential shortcomings should form the basis for a preventative substitution of missing nutrients or adaption of the vegan diet.

Plant proteins have a lower digestibility and a more limited amino acid composition than animal derived proteins. Therefore, their intake has to be increased by 30-35% for children up to the age of two years, by 20-30% for two to six year olds and by 15-20% for those older than six years of age to meet the required level. This will translate into an additional 2-14 g of protein per day. Children have higher requirements for essential amino acids, according to the 2007 WHO/FAO/UNU report.

To ensure a complete and sufficient essential amino acid supply, a well-planned mixture of different plant-derived proteins (e.g. cereals, nuts, seeds, fruits, legumes and vegetables) should be provided within 24 hours. Due to the higher bulk volume of plant protein in relation to gastral filling capacity, a premature feeling of satiety could lead to a possible energy deficit. Food with concentrated calories and nutrients such as mashed tofu or avocado, bean spreads and cooked dried fruits could be used in such a situation.

If an infant cannot be breastfed, the only adequate vegan alternative is a soy-based methionine-fortified infant formula, as recommended by the ESPGHAN Committee on Nutrition. There are no commercial formula options that do not contain animal products for those infants, who are intolerant to soy formula. Moreover, compared to infant formulas based on cow's milk, soy-based formulas have a higher concentration of phytate, aluminum, and phytoestrogens (isoflavones) which might have detrimental effects for the infant, unless these formulas have been specifically pretreated to decrease the concentration of these sub-stances. A recent systematic review concluded that modern soy-based infant formulas were safe regarding growth and bone health as well as metabolic, reproductive, endocrine, immune and neurological func-tions. Omega-3 fatty acids such as α-linolenic acid (ALA), eicosapentaenoic acid (EPA), and docosahex-aenoic acid (DHA) are essential for neurological development (e.g. synaptogenesis, retina development). As DHA and EPA are abundant in seafood and algae, a child not receiving these foods can only rely on precursors of DHA and EPA such as linolenic acid, which can be found in e.g. flaxseed, walnuts, rapeseed, chia6, Preterm children are at a higher risk of developing a deficiency in these nutrients, as their capacity to convert precursors is probably limited. Supplementation with long-chain n-3 fatty acids could be consid-ered, more research is needed.

Iron has an important role in hemoglobin synthesis, nerve myelination, neurotransmitter synthesis, and hippocampal energy metabolism. Iron requirements are higher during infant and adolescent growth spurts. Iron deficiency can contribute to anemia and more rarely to atrophic gastritis, which can lead to a decreased production of the intrinsic factor, which is necessary for vitamin B12 absorption. Children low on iron seem to score lower in developmental screening tests. Phytates, abundant in plant products, inhibit non-heme iron as well as zinc absorption by forming insoluble complexes in the gastroin-testinal tract. Iron from non-meat sources has due to its high content of phytates, dietary fibers and tannins a lower bioavailability. As long as our knowledge about phytoferritin is still limited children fed on a vegan diet should increase their iron intake by about 1.8 times, compared to those fed on animal products. Sufficient amount of vitamin C rich food can partly compensate for this decreased bioavailability of iron by reducing Fe^{3+} to the more soluble Fe^{2+}.

If zinc is not provided by animal products, it has to be supplied from fermented soy products (e.g. miso, tempeh), seeds and nuts6. As vegetarians and vegans have a high intake of phytates and polyphenols, zinc absorption is often diminished. However, data on zinc serum concentrations are sparse and difficult to cor-relate with dietary intake. Clinical signs of deficiency are rare among vegetarian and vegan children. According to the International Zinc Nutrition Consultative Group (IZiNCG), zinc should be supplemented (5 mg Zn/day for children aged 6–36 months, 10 mg Zn/day for older children) in case of a low dietary intake.

Vitamin D can be produced endogenously via skin exposure to ultraviolet light. However, the recommended minimum of 30 min/D on uncovered arms without applied sun screen is not always feasible or possible to follow (e.g. in winter). Vitamin D can also be obtained from dietary sources such as fatty fish and egg yolk for omnivores and mushrooms for vegetarians and vegans. Children with decreased dietary intake, lack of sun exposure or with a dark skin are at risk of a hypovitaminosis D and are encouraged to supplement with 600 IU of vitamin D3. The abstinence of milk and milk products in a vegan diet decreases the intake of calcium; this is relevant for infants after being weaned from breast milk or infant formulas. Vegetables low in oxalate such as broccoli, Chinese cabbage or collards are good sources of bioavailable calcium. Alternatively, calcium-fortified plant drinks, juices and calcium-rich mineral water are available. The FCN recom-mends a supplementation with 400 IU/day for every infant up to 1 year, regardless the type of nutrition and with 600 IU/D for toddlers up to 18 years. If this recommendation is followed, the risk of rickets or hy-pocalcemia is very low.

As with other micronutrients, the content of iodine in breast milk is dependent on the nutritional status of the mother. As seen in chapter 6.2 iodine is a critical micronutrient in an unsupplemented vegan diet. Low intakes during pregnancy and breastfeeding can exacerbate an iodine deficiency, in both mother and infant. Infants fed with formula milk receive the recommended daily supply of 80 µg per day. A risk of iodine deficiency can occur if they are solely fed with self-prepared food. To prevent a deficiency the FCN-publication "Nutrition in the last 1000 years" recommends partially replacing self-prepared food with iodine supplemented food or adding iodine supplementation of 50 µg per day.

As mentioned before, an unsupplemented vegan diet is lacking in vitamin B12.

A prolonged vitamin B12 deficiency will lead to a severe and potentially not fully reversible delay in the neuropsychological de-velopment of affected children. Vitamin B12 deficiency under a vegetarian diet (measured by MMA and holoTCII) has been reported for pregnant women (62%) and for children (25% - 86%)99. Breastfed infants will suffer from birth their mother's milk is low in vitamin B12, this is the reason we recommend to test the vitamin B12 status of the lactating mother. There are so far no studies we know giving evidence on the necessary quantity and time interval of orally supplied vitamin B12 to reach a physiologically adequate intra-cellular concentration, as shown by a normalized measurement of MMA. The recommended intake of vita-min B12 for breastfed vegan infants is 0.4 g/day during the first 4 month of life and 0.8 g/day, beginning at 5 months of age and should be increased up the recommended intake of 3.0 g/day for adolescents52. Because absorption of vitamin B12 is dose dependent saturated.

Different health associations state that well-balanced and planned vegetarian and vegan diets are compat-ible with a healthy upbringing and are appropriate at all stages of fetal, infant, child and adolescent growth. The focus on well-balanced and planned diets needs to be emphasized in all recommendations.

Ageing

No longitudinal prospective study was found monitoring very long-term vegan diets (including the assess-ment of specific dietary patterns and degree of adherence) and their impact on health. The consequences of long-term adherence to a vegan diet compared to the impact of a dietary switch to a vegan diet at a later stage of life have also not been investigated.

No specific vegan dietary recommendations have been made for an ageing population.

General nutrient recommendations for older adults are often higher than for healthy adults (<65 years old), some of the concerned nutrients are those, which are often at risk of deficiency in a vegan diet: protein, vitamin D, zinc, vitamin B12 and calcium. A vegan diet could therefore exacerbate nutritional deficiencies, which could be critical in the case of polymorbidity and frailty. In particular, protein recommendations for older adults following a vegan diet should be investigated, taking into account the higher needs at older ages (1.0-1.2 g/kg body weight) and the possible lower digestibility of plant proteins.

A matched cross-sectional study with institutionalized older adults, with 22 female and 7 male vegetarian (females: 84.1 ±5.1yrs, males: 80.5 ±7.5 yrs) and 23 female and 7 male bon-vegetarians (females: 84.3 ±5.0 yrs, males: 80.6 ±7.3 yrs) concluded that a vegetarian diet does not have a negative impact on the nutritional status and health indicators (blood profile, anthropometrics, handgrip strength).

A Taiwanese longitudinal study has several limitations, the main being the short duration of the longitudinal study (1 year), the other being the unknown number of older vegans in the cross-sectional part of the study. The metabolic profile of participants following a plant-based diet (vegan, lacto-vegetarian, ovo-lacto-vege-tarian) analysed in this study seems to be more favourable than that of omnivores in all age groups. Age itself is a risk factor for most non-communicable diseases.

Vegan diets and non-communicable diseases

In this chapter, the focus is on the impact of vegan diets on health, with the aim to assess whether a vegan diet is associated with an increased or decreased risk for major non-communicable diseases, such as over-weight /obesity, type 2 diabetes, cardiovascular diseases (CVD) and some cancer forms and other diseases. In the following chapters, the main results of recently published scientific studies are presented, based on vegan data, but including data on vegetarian diets, when these are compared to vegan diets. The evaluation of scientific evidence of the results was based on a grading system developed by the American Diabetes Association (ADA) to clarify and codify the evidence that forms the basis for the recommendations to im-prove health outcomes.

Overweight / Obesity

Prevention

Observational and case-control studies show that a long-term vegan diet is associated with a lower body weight than an omnivorous diet, no causality can be deducted from such studies. A follow-up study (EPIC-Oxford) over 5.3 years shows that a vegan diet does not prevent age-associated weight gain, how-ever, the annual weight gain is significantly lower in the vegan participants (males +284 g, females +303 g), compared to omnivores (males: +406 g, females +423 g). The mean age-adjusted BMI (kg/m2) increased from values of 22.6 to 23.2 (male vegans) and from 22.4 to 22.9 (female vegans), whereas omnivores had an initial mean age-adjusted BMI of 24.7 (males) and 23.8 (females), and increased to 25.3 and 24.8 re-spectively. In this study the vegan group had a lower mean energy intake (-279 kcal/day, compared to omnivores).

Age-adjusted mean body mass index (BMI) at baseline and follow-up by diet groups for men and women who were in the same diet group at both times.

Weight loss in overweight / obese subjects

The question thus arises, whether a vegan diet could be an effective weight loss strategy in overweight or obese subjects. Several systematic reviews and meta-analysis of mostly randomized controlled trials (RCT), in particular those of Huang et al. who selected studies according to Jadad et al. quality criteria and those of Barnard et al. have shown that a vegan diet can lead to significantly greater weight loss in comparison to their control (non-vegetarian) diet groups.

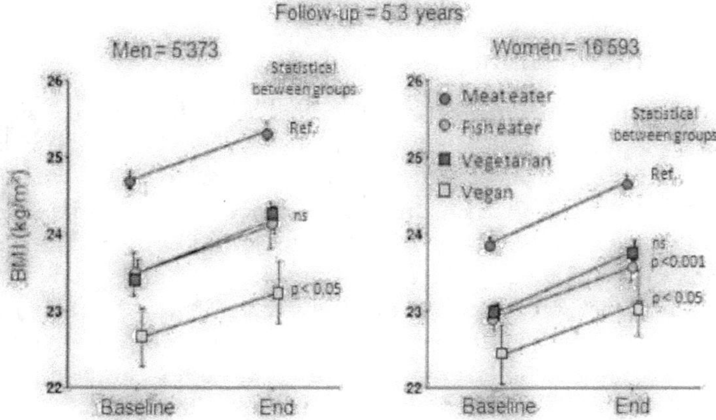

Pooled weighted mean differences in weight reduction observed intervention trials for vegan diets as compared to non-vegetarian diets.

However, these changes are not statistically different from other weight-loss diets reported in the recent systematic review and meta-analysis from Tobias et al. Studies included in this systematic review in-cluded energy-reduced omnivore diets, ovo-lacto-vegetarian diets, or Atkins diets.

Most of these studies have a high heterogeneity and are of a rather short duration in addition to other limitations that reduce their scientific evidence to the level C, based on the grading system developed by the American Diabetic Association. Therefore, long-term intervention trials are needed to investigate the effects of vegan and vegetarian diets, the caloric restriction on weight control and the cardiometabolic risk.

In conclusion, the data shows that there is no evidence that a vegan diet has a definite superiority in com-parison to a balanced diet for weight control or to weight loss diets recommended for overweight or obesity.

Type 2 diabetes

The role of nutrition and other life-style factors in the prevention and treatment of type 2 diabetes (T2DM) has been recognised. There is good evidence (grade A) of the impact of a balanced energy intake and weight loss (-5% of body weight), as well as B-grade evidence for diets with fruit and pulses as the main carbohydrate sources that are rich in fibres. These are elements of a well-planned vegan diet. Therefore, recent epidemiological literature was screened in order to evaluate the impact of a self-chosen vegan diet on the risk of T2DM (preventive effects) and the efficacy of a vegan diet as a nutritional therapeutic ap-proach.

Prevention

A case-control study was performed by Tonstad et al. with the Adventist Health Study-2 (SDA) cohort, with 60'903 participants. The data were corrected for 10 factors, including age, sex, physical activity and BMI. The ensuing results showed that the odds ratio (OR) for the prevalence of self-declared T2DM was 0.51 for vegans (CI 0.40 - 0.66), 0.54 for ovo-lacto-vegetarians (CI 0.49 - 0.60), 0.70 for pesco-vegetarians (CI 0.61 - 0.80), and 0.76 for semi-vegetarians (CI 0.40 - 0.66), when compared to the reference group (omnivores). Furthermore, in a subgroup of 42'017 participants in this SDA cohort, the same authors reported after a follow-up of two years, a lower incidence of T2DM for vegans (0.54%), for ovo-lacto-vegetar-ians (1.08%), for pesco-vegetarians (1.29%), and semi-vegetarians (0.92%), when compared to the omni-vores (2.12%, p<0.001). However, as indicated by the authors, a number of study limitations must be considered when interpreting these findings.

Two cross-sectional studies, performed in Asian countries, have contradictory results; these studies were therefore not further taken into account in this review, due to the different dietary and lifestyle patterns.

A direct comparison with other lifestyle and dietary choices, which have shown a protective effect (e.g. Mediterranean diet) is still lacking, therefore vegan diets are not specifically recommended to delay T2DM.

Therapy

For their systematic review, Yokoyama et al. found only 6 intervention studies fulfilling the criteria established by the "Cochrane Handbook for Systematic Reviews Intervention"11 among the studies published between 1947 and 2013. Vegan diets (N=4) and lacto-vegetarian (N=1) were compared to control diets, using the glycated hemoglobin A1c (HbA1c) measurements as the outcome. Of the 5 studies with 258 diabetic participants included for 12 to 74 weeks (mean = 28 weeks), three were randomized, two were non-randomized comparisons, and one was a cluster randomized trial. In the pooled analysis, con-sumption of vegan diets was associated with a significant mean reduction in HbA1c (-0.39% 95% CI: -0.62 to -0.15; P=0.001; I^2 = 3.0; P for heterogeneity = 0.389), compared to non-vegetarian diets.

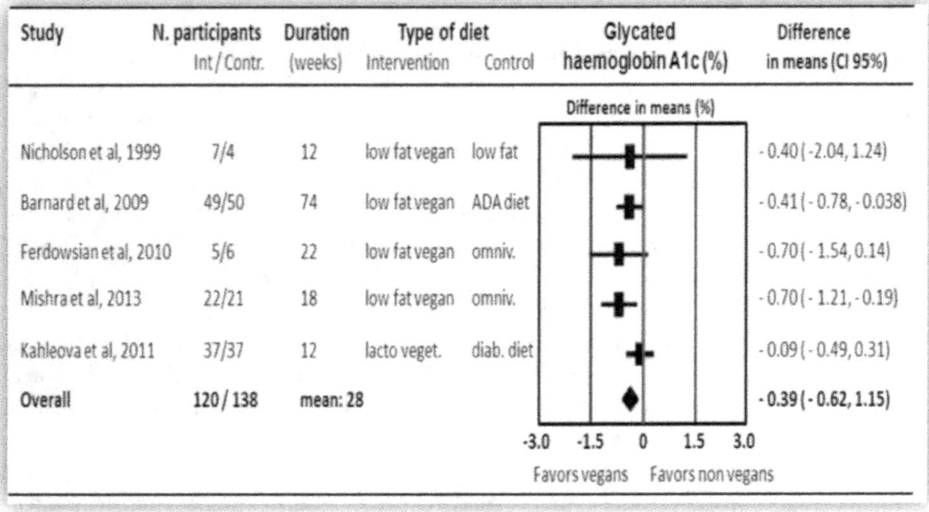

Pooled mean changes in glycated hemoglobin A1c level in response to the vegan and vegetarian diet as compared to other control diets in type 2 diabetes

The corresponding mean reduction in fasting blood glucose levels was not significant (–0.36 mmol/l; 95% CI:-1.04 to 0.32; P = 0.301; I^2 = 0; P for heterogeneity = 0.710). In this analysis, consumption of vegetarian diets was associated with significant mean differences in energy intake (–139.8 kcal; 95% CI: –232.8 to - 46.7; P= 0.003) as well as for the other macronutrients. The magnitude of the effect size is approximately one-half of that seen with metformin, which is used as first-line oral therapy for elevated HbA1c levels.

A further systematic review on the same topic was conducted by Ajala et al. providing a succinct but robust evidence base to guide clinicians and patients on the most suitable dietary intervention to improve glycemic control. 16 RCTs were included (n = 3'073 in the final analysis across 3'460 randomly assigned individuals). Compared with their respective control diets, a greater improvement in HbA1c reductions was observed for Mediterranean diet (-0.47%, p< 0.00001, I2= 82%, N= 3) than for low carbohydrate (-0.12%, P=0.04, I2 = 75%, N= 8), for low-glycemic index (-0.14% P = 0.008, I2= 80%, N= 3) or high-protein diets (-0.28%, P < 0.00001, I2= 60%, N= 2). Low-carbohydrate and Mediterranean diets led to greater weight loss (-0.69 kg, P = 0.21, and -1.84 kg, P < 0.00001, respectively).

For the only vegan RCT reported in the Ajala review (by Barnard et al.), a significant reduction in HbA1c was achieved in comparison to the diabetic diet recommended by the American Diabetic Association, when the effects were assessed before the medication changes (-0.41%, P= 0.03). The changes were however non-significant (-0.20%, P=0.43) when reported for the intention-to-treat analysis.

According to the review of the existing literature, Ajala et al. therefore consider that low-carbohydrate, low–glycemic index, Mediterranean, and high protein diets are effective in improving glycemic control and should be therefore considered in the overall strategy of T2DM management, but no specific recommenda-tions are given for the vegan/vegetarian diets.

Finally, Emadian et al. conducted a recent systematic review of eleven RCTs, including the only vegan trial from Barnard et al. in order to assess the effects of various dietary interventions on glycemic control in overweight and obese adults with T2DM, when adjusted for weight loss. Overall, they conclude, "there is currently insufficient evidence to suggest that any particular diet is superior in treating overweight and obese patients with T2DM ". However, although the Mediterranean, vegan and low-GI diets appear to be promis-ing, these authors consider that "further research that controls for weight loss and the effects of diabetes medications in larger samples is needed.

In conclusion, given the limited number of studies with sufficient methodological quality providing a low level of scientific evidence (C), new findings are required to assert that vegan diets offer more advantages than non-VGT for the metabolic control of type 2 diabetes.

Cardiovascular diseases

Today, cardiovascular diseases (CVD), such as ischemic heart disease (IHD) and stroke significantly in-crease the burden of disease in Switzerland. They cause premature deaths and CVD morbidity contributes to the rising costs in the health sector. In 2014, CVD were the first cause of mortality as well in women (34%) as in men (31%). Among CVD deaths, 78% were due to cardiac origin, namely IHD and myocardial infarction, and 16.5 % to strokes. Therefore CVD have been included in National Strategy for the Prevention of Non-communicable diseases 2017–2024.

Risk factors for cardiovascular diseases

Dietary habits influence the CVD risk, either by effecting risk factors such as blood pressure, cholesterol, body weight and diabetes, or through other effects. Healthy dietary practices have been recommended as a cornerstone of CVD prevention in all individuals for decades. In the last decade, plant-based dietary patterns have become a popular recommendation, due to a variety of reported health benefits to overall health and to cardiovascular (CV) risk and disease in particular. However, most evidence on the rela-tion between nutrition and CVD is based on observational studies; randomized clinical trials estimating the impact of diet on clinical endpoints are scarce. The aim of this chapter is to highlight scientific knowledge concerning the influence of vegan diets on CV risk factors and CVD morbidity and mortality, namely is-chemic heart disease (IHD) and cerebrovascular disease (CerVD).

Hypertension

The main diet-related determinants of hypertension are high salt intake, obesity and excess alcohol con-sumption. Western vegetarians have a lower average BMI than non-vegetarians, but do not necessarily have low intakes of salt and alcohol. To examine the association between vegan and vegetarian diets and blood pressure, Yokoyama et al. conducted a systematic review and meta-analysis. Of the 258 studies identified, 32 observational studies and 7 clinical controlled trials met the inclusion criteria. In the 32 observational cross-sectional studies (total n=21'604 participants; mean age 46.6 years), consumption of vegetarian diets was also associated with both a significantly lower mean systolic BP (−6.9 mmHg; 95% CI: -9.1 to -4.7; P < 0.001, I2 = 91.4 P< 0.001 for heterogeneity) and with a lower diastolic BP (-4.7 mmHg; 95% CI: -6.3 to -3.1; P < 0.001, I2 = 92.6 P< 0.001 for heterogeneity) compared with the consumption of omniv-orous diets. A significant reduction of systolic BP (-28 to -4.9 mmHg) was also observed in the four vegan studies. However, due to the wide heterogeneity of these results and the multiple limitations of such studies, the scientific evidence for the anti-hypertensive effects of vegan and vegetarian diets must be considered as low (C).

Yokoyama et al. also performed a meta-analysis of the seven clinical controlled trials, with 311 participants (mean age 44.5 years), mainly without hypertension. The consumption of vegetarian (N= 5) or vegan (N= 2) diets was associated with a significant reduction in mean systolic BP (-4.8 mm Hg; 95% CI: -6.6 to -3.1; P < 0.001, I2 = 0, P = 0.45) and diastolic BP (-2.2 mmHg; 95% CI: -3.5 to -1.0; P < 0.001, I2 = 0, P = 0.43), compared to omnivorous diets. The magnitude of the anti-hypertensive effect was less pronounced here than in the observational studies. Moreover, the changes in systolic and diastolic BP were significant only in the oldest of five vegetarian trials.

Sources	N of participants	Mean baseline Blood pressure	Duration (weeks)	Type of diets Intervention	Control	Blood pressure (mmHg)	Difference in means (mmHg, 95% CI)	P value
Systolic blood pressure						Difference in mean changes (%)		
Rouse et al, 1983	38	127.7	6	Ovo-lacto	Omnivorous		−6.8 (−9.6 to −4.0)	<0.001
Ferdowsian et al, 2010	113	117.8	22	Vegan	Omnivorous		−5.7 −11.1 −0.3	0.04
Margetts et al, 1986	39	155.4	6	Ovo-lacto	Omnivorous		−3.5 −6.9 −0.1	0.047
Hakala & Karvetti, 1989	73	129.9	52	Lacto	Omnivorous		−3.3 −8.3 1.8	0.21
Kestin et al, 1989	17	128.0	6	Ovo-lacto	Omnivorous		−3.0 −9.1 3.1	0.34
Sciarrone et al, 1993	20	134.2	6	Ovo-lacto	Omnivorous		+1.5 −15.3 18.3	0.86
Nicholson et al, 1999	11	141.3	12	Vegan	Omnivorous		+8.5 −10.2 27.2	0.37
Overall	**311**	mean = 15.7					**−4.8 −6.6 −3.1**	**<0.001**
(Heterogeneity : I^{22} = 0.0; P = 0.45)								
Diastolic blood pressure								
Ferdowsian et al, 2010	113	79.7	22	Vegan	Omnivorous		−5.5 −9.1 −1.9	<0.003
Rouse et al, 1983	38	76.4	6	Ovo-lacto	Omnivorous		−2.7 −4.7 −0.7	<0.008
Hakala & Karvetti, 1989	73	85.0	52	Lacto	Omnivorous		−2.5 −9.2 4.2	0.46
Margetts et al, 1986	39	99.9	6	Ovo-lacto	Omnivorous		−1.2 −3.1 0.7	0.22
Sciarrone et al, 1993	20	77.2	6	Ovo-lacto	Omnivorous		−1.0 −14.8 12.8	0.89
Kestin et al, 1989	17	79.0	6	Ovo-lacto	Omnivorous		−0.8 −6.0 4.4	0.76
Nicholson et al, 1999	11	84.7	12	Vegan	Omnivorous		+4.8 −8.3 17.9	0.47
Overall	**311**	mean = 15.7					**−2.2 −3.5 −1.0**	**<0.001**
(Heterogeneity : I^{22} = 0.0; P = 0.43)								

Axis: -30 -15 0 15 30

Favors vegetarians   Favors omnivores

Pooled systolic and diastolic blood pressure responses to vegan and vegetarian diets in clinical trials

However, diverging results were observed between the two vegan trials. Due to several signif-icant limitations of these controlled trials such as small sample size, short duration and lack of adjustment for confounding factors, only C-grade of evidence can be attributed to this meta-analysis. As concluded by these authors, "despite consumption of vegetarian diets is associated with lower BP, further studies are required to clarify which types of vegetarian diets are most strongly associated with lower BP". Overall, these effect sizes are similar to those observed with commonly recommended lifestyle modifications, such as adoption of a low-sodium diet or a weight reduction of 5kg, and are approximately half the magnitude of those observed with pharmaceutical therapy, such as administration of angiotensin-converting enzyme in-hibitors to individuals with hypertension.

Dyslipidemia

Theoretically, in comparison with omnivorous diets, vegan and vegetarian diets may have a beneficial effect on the blood lipid profile, due to the lower intake of saturated fats as well as the high fibre intake.

Several cross-sectional studies have shown that concentrations of TC, LDL-C, and TG were lower in vege-tarians than in omnivores.

A recent systematic review and meta-analysis of the published RCTs was conducted by Wang et al. to comprehensively assess the overall effects of vegetarian diets on blood lipids. Among these 10 studies, 6 included a vegan diet, 2 included a ovo-lacto-vegetarian diet, and 2 included a lacto-vegetarian diet, with a total of 774 participants treated by the diet during 3 weeks to 18 months (median = 12 weeks). In these trials, a majority of recruited patients were diabetics or with BMI > 25 kg/m² and some were receiving lipid-lowering agents. The results provide evidence that vegetarian diets significantly lower the mean blood con-centrations of total cholesterol, LDL-cholesterol and HDL-cholesterol (pooled estimated changes were - 0.36 mmol/l, P<0.001, -0.34 mmol/l, P < 0.001, and -0.10 mmol/l, P < 0.001 respectively), without affecting triglyceride levels. Moderate to high heterogeneity of the results was detected for total cholesterol (I^2 = 53.5 %) and LDL-cholesterol (I^2 = 72.4%).

The observed reduction in cholesterol levels was significant in 2 of 4 vegetarian diet studies. Among the 6 vegan studies, the estimated changes in cholesterol ranged from -0.78 to 0 mmol/l, and were significant only in two older studies: - 0.54 mmol/l, CI 95%: -0.94 to -0.14 and -0.78 mmol/l, CI 95%: -1.34, to - 0.57187.

Again, the studies included in this meta-analysis suffer from several limitations acknowledged by the authors and consequently reduce the level of the scientific evidence (C). Moreover, the evidence that these changes in lipid profile induced vegetarian diets preventing CVD is still lacking. By comparison, available evidence exists for the dietary patterns such as the Mediterranean diet, which has been more extensively evaluated and has been proven to be effective to reduce CV risk factors, as well as to contributing to CVD prevention.

Study	N. of participants	Diet	Design	Duration (weeks/months)	Total cholesterol (mmol/L)	Weighted mean difference (mmol/l, 95% CI)
					Weighted mean difference (mmol/L, 95% CI)	
Cooper et al, 1982,	15	Lacto	CO	3 wk		- 0.51 (-0.94 to -0.08)
Kestin et al, 1989	26	Ovo-lacto	CO	6 wk		- 0.61 (-1.14 to -0.08)
Ling et al, 1992	18	Vegan	PL	4 wk		- 0.77 (-1.92 to -0.38)
Nicholson et al, 1999	11	Vegan	PL	12 wk		- 0.00 (-1.05 to 1.05)
Barnard et al, 2000	35	Vegan	CO	2 mo		- 0.54 (- 0.94 to - 0.14)
Agren et al, 2001	29	Vegan	PL	3 mo		- 0.78 (- 1.34 to -0.57)
Burke et al, 2007	176	Ovo-lacto	PL	18 mo		- 0.18 (- 0.57 to 0.21)
Barnard et al, 2009	58	Vegan	PL	12 mo		- 0.18 (- 0.57 to 0.21)
Kahleova et al, 2011	99	Lacto	PL	74 wk		- 0.17 (- 0.46 to 0.12)
Mishra et al, 2013	291	Vegan	PL	12 wk		- 0.21 (- 0.44 to 0.02)
Overall (Heterogeneity: I^2 = 53.5%)				median = 12 wk		- 0.36 (- 0.55 to - 0.17)

Design: PL = parallel groups, CO = cross-over

Favors vegetarians   Favors omnivores

5 Effects of vegetarian diets on total cholesterol concentrations as compared to omnivorous diets in Interventional trials.

Cardiovascular diseases

A collaborative analysis of five prospective studies, by Key and al., is frequently reported in the literature. This study showed that mortality from IHD was 26% lower in vegans (RR 0.74, 95% CI: 0.46 - 1.21), 34% than for vegetarians (RR 0.66, CI: 0.52 - 0.83, significant), both when compared to omnivores. These older results were based on observational studies that suffered from key limitations. More solid evidence is nec-essary before making recommendations for the general population. Therefore, the following chapter aims to summarize the scientific literature established up to the end of January 2018 in order to confirm the possible contribution of vegan or vegetarian diets to reduce the risk of CVD, including IHD and strokes.

Prevention of Cardiovascular diseases

To examine whether vegan and vegetarian diets, as compared to non-vegetarian diets, are associated with reduced incidence of a first CV event, Crowe et al. have analyzed the risk of hospitalization following the incidence of non-fatal or fatal IHD events among 44'561 men and women involved in the EPIC–Oxford study. After an average follow-up of 11.6 years, vegetarians (including vegans) had a 32% lower risk (95% CI: 0.58 - 0.81) of IHD events than did non-vegetarians, when adjusted for age, smoking, alcohol, physical activity, educational level, and Townsend Deprivation Index and use of oral contraceptives or hormone therapy for menopause in women. This rate was only slightly attenuated, but remained significant, after additional adjustment of BMI. When this analysis was stratified by sex a significant risk reduction of IHD events of -26% (95% CI: 0.58 - 0.95) in both men and women (-36%; 95% CI: 0.51 - 0.81) was observed.

No specific analysis was performed here to examine whether vegan diets might be associated with similar benefits for CerVD or CVD in general.

The data reported by Christiansen al. issue from a cohort comprising 6'532 members of the Danish Sev-enth-day Adventist Church (SDA) and another cohort totalizing 3'720 Baptists followed in the Danish Na-tional Patient Register from 1977 to 2009. The SDA advocates against alcohol consumption and tobacco smoking and recommends an ovo-lacto-vegetarian diet, but no specifically a vegan diet. In addition, mem-bers of SDA were expected to be physically active and have stable social relationships. Members of the Baptist community were encouraged not to smoke or drink alcohol.

During the 12-year follow-up, compared with the general Danish population, the SDA members experienced a standardized incidence ratio of a first IHD that was significantly lower in women (-9%; 95% CI: 0.83 - 0.99), but not in men (-8%; 95% CI: 0.83 - 1.03). For a first CerVD this ratio was not significantly lower neither in women (-3%; 95% CI: 0.88 - 1.08) nor in men (-7%; 95% CI: 0.81 - 1.06).

Similar trends were obtained among the Baptists, with a significant lower incidence ratio of IHD in women (-22%; 95% CI: 0.69 - 0.89) but not in men (-3%; 95% CI: 0.86-1.10), while the ratio for CerVD was not significantly reduced, either in women (-6%; 95% CI: 0.82 - 1.07) or in men (-8%; 95% CI: 0.79 - 1.08). Whether similar results could be obtained by vegan diets needs to be determined. Concerning the key limitations of this observational study, namely the lack of adjustment for confounding factors, caution is needed when interpreting these results.

In summary, according to the very small number of studies available to date (two Danish studies, one EPIC-Oxford), and to the limitations of such observational studies, the scientific evidence in favour of vegetarian diets for the primary prevention of CVD is low (level C of evidence). Nevertheless, the results reported here show that vegetarian diets are associated with a significant reduction in the risk of hospitalization for a first IHD in women, but not clearly in men, and with a non-significant reduction for CerVD. Whether vegan diets may have similar effects has not yet been demonstrated. Further research is clearly required to prove the potential benefits of vegan and vegetarian diets for the primary prevention of CVD.

Cardiovascular Diseases Mortality

The review of scientific literature published between 2007 and January 2018 identified three systematic reviews of relevant prospective cohort studies evaluating the link between the vegetarian diets and the risk of CV mortality.

The first systematic review and meta-analysis of Huang et al. incorporated seven prospective cohort studies of which three were already included in the series of Key et al. published in 1999. Among a total of 124'706 participants recruited between 1955 and 1999 and followed during 10 to 23 years, the IHD mor-tality was significantly lower (-29%; 95% CI: 0.56 - 0.87; $I^2 = 31\%$) in vegetarians and vegans than in non-vegetarians. However, this association was neither significant for CerVD mortality (-12%, 95% CI: 0.70 - 1.06; $I^2 = 31\%$), nor for circulatory diseases mortality (-16%, 95% CI: 0.54 - 1.14; $I^2 = 58\%$).

Kwok et al. carried out the second systematic review and meta-analysis of eight prospective cohort stud-ies. Among them, the cohort of Adventist Health Study-2 was added to the 7 cohorts included by Huang et al. but with different sample sizes and follow-ups. Their objectives were firstly to update the current un-derstanding of the lower risk of CV mortality associated with vegetarian diets (pesco-, semi-, ovo-lacto and vegans) compared to non-vegetarian diets. A second objective was to determine whether the positive find-ings could be specific to the vegetarian diets alone or to the healthier lifestyles observed among the members of the cohort of the Seventh Day Adventists Church, by comparison to other cohort studies. Seven cohort studies were included in this pooled analysis to obtain a level of quality deemed to be moderate in five studies and low to moderate in 2 studies. In addition to the lack of collected data, there were also differences in the use of adjustments for confounders such as weight, smoking and alcohol in vegetarian studies.

3 SDA studies showed a significant mean reduction of IHD mortality (- 40%; 95% CI: 0.43 - 0.80). The non-SDA studies confirm this risk reduction, but to a lesser extent (-16 % for the pooled results; 95% CI 0.74 - 0.96, I2 = 0%, P = 0.92). When combining the SDA and non-SDA groups, the risk reduction was -29% (95% CI: 0.57 - 0.87; I2 = 83%. This risk reduction associated with vegetarian diets was significant in men (-19%; 95% CI: 0.68 - 0.97) and near to the statistical signifi-cance in women (-26%; 95% CI: 0.54 - 1.01), with a large heterogeneity (I2 = 88%, P = 0.0002) of the results, as compared to with the mean of the 4 non-SDA studies: (-16 %; 95% CI 0.74 - 0.96, I2 = 0%, P = 0.92).

For CerVD mortality, the risk reduction pooled for the two SDA studies was 29% (95% CI 0.41 - 1.20; I2 = 83%), but again with a high heterogeneity of these results. In contrast, no significant differences were found in any of the four non-SDA studies, nor in the mean risk of CerVD (+5%; 95% CI: 0.89 - 1.24). However, when SDA and non-SDA studies were pooled, there was a small and non-significant reduction in relative risk (-7%; 95% CI: 0.70 - 1.23); I2 = 79%). In this meta-analysis, no data were provided for overall CV mortality.

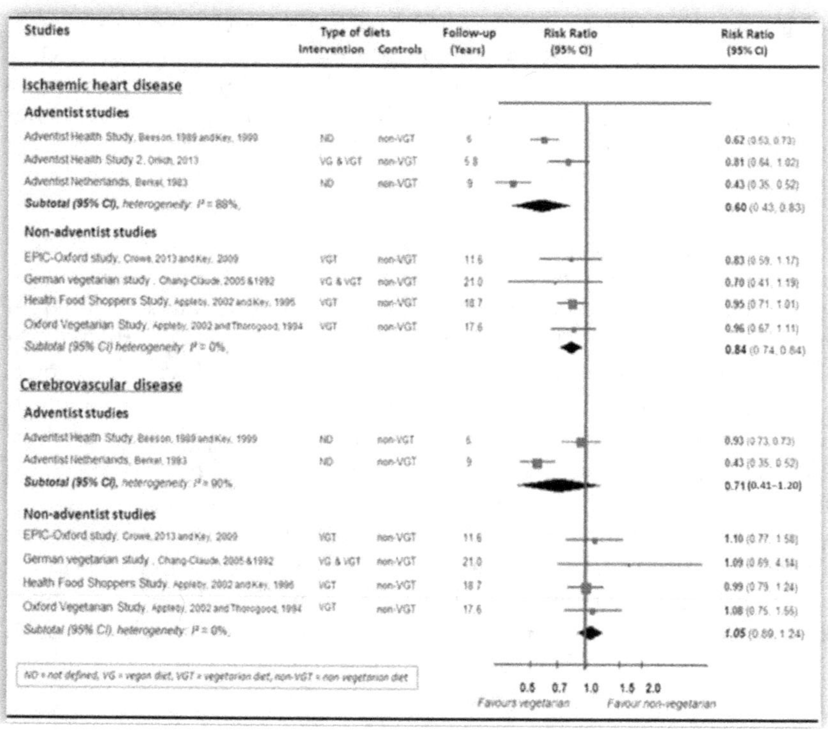

Studies	Type of diets Intervention	Controls	Follow-up (Years)	Risk Ratio (95% CI)	Risk Ratio (95% CI)
Ischaemic heart disease					
Adventist studies					
Adventist Health Study, Beeson, 1989 and Key, 1999	ND	non-VGT	6		0.62 (0.53, 0.73)
Adventist Health Study 2, Orlich, 2013	VG & VGT	non-VGT	5.8		0.81 (0.64, 1.02)
Adventist Netherlands, Berkel, 1983	ND	non-VGT	9		0.43 (0.35, 0.52)
Subtotal (95% CI), heterogeneity: I^2 = 88%,					**0.60 (0.43, 0.83)**
Non-adventist studies					
EPIC-Oxford study, Crowe, 2013 and Key, 2009	VGT	non-VGT	11.6		0.83 (0.59, 1.17)
German vegetarian study, Chang-Claude, 2005 & 1992	VG & VGT	non-VGT	21.0		0.70 (0.41, 1.19)
Health Food Shoppers Study, Appleby, 2002 and Key, 1996	VGT	non-VGT	18.7		0.95 (0.71, 1.01)
Oxford Vegetarian Study, Appleby, 2002 and Thorogood, 1994	VGT	non-VGT	17.6		0.96 (0.67, 1.11)
Subtotal (95% CI) heterogeneity: I^2 = 0%,					**0.84 (0.74, 0.84)**
Cerebrovascular disease					
Adventist studies					
Adventist Health Study, Beeson, 1989 and Key, 1999	ND	non-VGT	6		0.93 (0.73, 0.73)
Adventist Netherlands, Berkel, 1993	ND	non-VGT	9		0.43 (0.35, 0.52)
Subtotal (95% CI), heterogeneity: I^2 = 90%,					**0.71 (0.41-1.20)**
Non-adventist studies					
EPIC-Oxford study, Crowe, 2013 and Key, 2009	VGT	non-VGT	11.6		1.10 (0.77, 1.58)
German vegetarian study, Chang-Claude, 2005 & 1992	VG & VGT	non-VGT	21.0		1.09 (0.69, 4.14)
Health Food Shoppers Study, Appleby, 2002 and Key, 1996	VGT	non-VGT	18.7		0.99 (0.79, 1.24)
Oxford Vegetarian Study, Appleby, 2002 and Thorogood, 1994	VGT	non-VGT	17.6		1.08 (0.75, 1.56)
Subtotal (95% CI), heterogeneity: I^2 = 0%,					**1.05 (0.89, 1.24)**

Meta-analysis of vegetarian diets and risk of death by ischaemic heart disease and cerebrovascular disease cohorts as compared to non-vegetarian diets, stratified by Seventh-Day Adventist and non-Adventist cohorts.

Overall, these data supporting the benefits of vegetarian diets are derived mainly from SDA studies that have different lifestyles and other factors that are not generalizable to the wider population. A similar point of view is given by Kwok et al. which concludes that "the reduction in IHD and all-cause mortality with vegetarian diet stems mainly from the Adventist studies, and there is much less convincing evidence from studies conducted in other populations. Once the SDA studies have been excluded, the results are either less significant or with a lesser magnitude of benefit, and this raises the concern that the non-dietary factors (confounders) in SDA lifestyle may be responsible for the risk reduction among the vegetarian studies. In addition, among men there appears to be greater benefit of vegetarian diet compared to women. In view of these inconsistent findings, we conclude that the benefits of vegetarian diet for reducing death and vascular events remain unproven."

A third recent systematic review with meta-analysis performed by Dinu et al. included a pool of three SDA and four non-SDA cohort studies, among them six were already analysed by Kwok et al. In comparison to omnivorous diets, vegetarian diets were associated with a significant reduction of IHD mortality (-25%; 95% Cl: 0.68 - 0.82, P < 0.001, I2 = 35%); but not with a significant one on the reduction of mortality from CerVD (-7%, 95% CI: 0.78 - 1.10; P = 0.39, I2 = 44%) or from CV mortality (-7%, 95% CI: 0.86 - 1.00, P = 0.07, I2 = 0%).

Similar limitations to that expressed by Kwok et al here above, need to be taken into account for the interpretation of the potential benefits of vegetarian diets on the CV risk.

It should be noted that the authors of these three meta-analyses did not perform a subgroup analysis specific to vegans. Consequently, the existing data do not permit a clarification of whether the benefits of vegan diets on CV mortality could be similar to those observed with vegetarian diets.

Nevertheless, in order to attempt to determine the influence of a vegan diet on the risk of mortality attributed to CVD, the results observed in two prospective cohort studies published in 2013 (Orlich, SDA) and in 2016 (Appleby, non-SDA) are clinically relevant.

The Adventist Health Study-2 (n=73'308, follow-up = 5.6 yr.), strong diverging results were obtained for the total CVD and IHD mortality risks between men and women following vegan diets, with men showing a significant decrease, whereas a non-significant risk increase was observed among women.

A vegan diet is associated with a significant lower mortality risk (CVD and IHD), when compared to other vegetarian diets in men. Very diverging results are observed in women, both when compared with men, but also when comparing the different diets. For the whole group (men and women pooled), a vegan diet is not associated with a more favourable outcome than other diets.

Hazard ratio for overall cardiovascular and specifically IHD mortality as a function of the type of vegetarian diet in comparison to omnivores of the "Adventist Health Study 2"

	Women (n= 48'203)		Men (n= 25'105)		Total women and men	
	CVD total	IHD	CVD total	IHD	CVD	IHD
Vegans (n= 5'548)	+ 18%, ns (CI 95%: 0.88 - 1.60)	+ 39%, ns (CI 95%: 0.87 - 2.24)	- 42%, s (CI 95%: 0.38 - 0.89)	- 55%, s (CI 95%: 0.21 - 0.94)	- 9%, ns (CI 95%: 0.71 - 1.16)	- 10%, ns (CI 95%: 0.60 - 1.33)
Ovo-lacto-vegetarians (n=21'177)	- 1%, ns (CI 95%: 0.81 - 1.22)	- 15%, ns (CI 95%: 0.59 - 1.22)	- 23%, s (CI 95%: 0.59 - 0.99)	- 24%, ns (CI 95%: 0.52 - 1.12)	- 10%, ns (CI 95%: 0.76 - 1.06)	- 18%, ns (CI 95%: 0.62 - 1.06)
Pesco-vegetarians (n=7'194)	- 10%, ns (CI 95%: 0.66 - 1.23)	- 49%, s (CI 95%: 0.26 - 0.99)	- 34%, s (CI 95%: 0.44 - 0.98)	- 23%, ns (CI 95%: 0.43 - 1.30)	- 20%, ns (CI 95%: 0.62 - 1.03)	- 35%, s (CI 95%: 0.43 - 0.97)
Semi-vegetarians (n=4'031)	- 7%, ns (CI 95%: 0.64 - 1.34)	+ 9%, ns (CI 95%: 0.60 - 1.98)	- 25%, ns (CI 95%: 0.43 - 1.32)	- 27%, ns (CI 95%: 0.33 - 1.60)	- 15%, ns (CI 95%: 0.63 - 1.16)	- 8%, ns (CI 95%: 0.57 - 1.51)
Total Vegetarians (n= 37'950)	- 1%, ns (CI 95%: 0.83 - 1.18)	- 12%, ns (CI 95%: 0.65 - 1.20)	- 29% s (CI 95% 0.57 - 0.90)	- 29% s (CI 95% 0.51 - 1.00)	- 13%, ns (CI 95%: 0.75 - 1.01)	- 19%, ns (CI 95%: 0.64 - 1.02)

Analyses of mortality were performed using Cox proportional hazards regression adjusted for different age, sex and race. Statistical significance: s = significant (in boldface), ns: not significant.

The analysis of both Oxford Vegetarian Study and EPIC-Oxford study performed by Apple by et al., (n=60'310, follow-up > 15 y.), vegans (men and women combined) have a non-significant slight decreased hazard ratio for IHD mortality (-10%, non-significant) among vegans when com-pared to non-vegetarian diets, as also seen with the Adventist study. When comparing the results between the two studies it is apparent that several results are in discordance, both in the risk tendency and the significance.

These diverging findings could be explained largely by the non-comparable lifestyles and dietary habits practiced by the various dietary groups of the American Adventist cohort and those of the two British cohorts, but are compatible with the meta-analysis by Kwock et al.

The non-significant risk increases observed in the British cohorts for CerVD and CVD mortality, for vegan and some other vegetarian diets, are in contradiction with the frequently reported significant benefits of a vegan / vegetarian diets.

Hazard ratio of cardiovascular mortality according to the type of vegetarian diet compared to non-vegetarian diets of the "Oxford Vegetarian Study & the EPIC-Oxford Cohort

	Ischaemic Heart disease	Cerebrovascular disease	Cardiovascular disease
Vegans	- 10%, ns	+ 61%, ns	+ 21%, ns
(n = 2'228)	(CI 95% : 0.53 - 1.55)	(CI 95% : 0.97 - 2.69)	(CI 95% : 0.88 - 1.66)
Pesco-vegetarians	+ 6%, ns	+ 36%, ns	+ 26%, s
(n = 8'516)	(CI 95% : 0.79 - 1.42)	(CI 95% : 0.99 - 1.87)	(CI 95% 1.05 - 1.51)
Semi-vegetarians (n =	-4%, ns	- 12%, ns	-2%, ns

Estimated by Cox Proportional hazards ratio regression adjusted for different risk factors. Statistical significance: s: significant, ns: not significant

The data presented in these different systematic reviews and meta-analyses of observational studies suggest that vegan and vegetarian diets could be associated with a lower risk of IHD mortality, but possibly not in vegan women.

Further investigation is needed, before recommending such types of diets for the general population, as a CVD preventive measure, in particular for women. In fact, the current scientific evidence does not support the favourable statements published recently to promote vegetarian and vegan diets. In addition, it should be noted that vegan diets are not specifically listed in the recommendations for the prevention and management of cardiovascular diseases and their risk factors on this topic by different authors involved in the Physicians Committee for Responsible Medicine promoting vegetarian and vegan diets.

Cancer

Approximately 20'800 men and 17'650 women develop cancer each year. Cancers of prostate, breast, colorectal and lung account for slightly more than half of the cases. Moreover, cancers are not only the second cause of death but they represent also the greatest number of years of potential life lost through death before 70 years of age. Although there are multiple causes of cancer, the scientific literature considers that there is an increased risk of the most frequent cancers such as breast, prostate, and colon in connection with body fat excess, high consumption of red and processed meats and alcohol. Conversely, a diet high in fiber, fruits and vegetables could have a pro-tective effect. Consequently, the recommendations of the Swiss League against Cancer advocate a bal-anced diet, rich in fruits and vegetables and poor in animal foods. The aim of this review is to update scientific knowledge on the influence of vegan diets on cancer prevention between 2007 and December 2017.

Cancer incidence

During the last decade, only Dinu et al. have performed a systematic review and a meta-analysis, which included cross-sectional and cohort studies, to evaluate the association between vegan or vegetarian diets and cancer incidence resp. mortality. With regard to incidence of total cancer, meta-analytic pooling under a random-effects model showed a significant lower risk of cancer among vegans (-15%; 95% CI: 0.75 - 0.95) and among vegetarians (-8%; 95% CI: 0.87 - 0.98) in comparison to omnivorous diets.

In the meta-analysis of Huang T et al., combined vegetarian and vegan diets were also associated with a significant lower risk of all-cancer (-18%; 95% CI: 0.67 - 0.97; I^2 = 27%) when pooling 7 prospective cohort studies, but the relative risk varied from -50% to + 12% in these studies.

To further examine the potential benefits of vegan diets on cancer incidence the results of the 5 large pro-spective cohort studies were published between 2007 and 2017, also presents also a comparison between the differences in incidence of all-cancer and site-specific cancers, by type of diet and gender Overall, vegans experienced modest risk reductions of incidence of all-cancer, either in the Adventist Health Study 2 (-14%; 95% CI: 0.73 - 1.00) or in the Oxford Vegetarian Study & EPIC-Oxford Cohort (-18%; 95% CI: 0.68 - 1.00). No significant association was found between a vegan diet and the different specific cancer sites. For colon-rectum cancer conflicting results were observed between the Adventist Health Study 2 (-14%; 95% CI: 0.59 - 1.24) and the Oxford Vegetarian Study & EPIC-Oxford Cohort (+31%; 95% CI: 0.82 - 2.11). In addition, in this later cohort study vegans have shown a significant higher risk of incidence of urinary tract cancers (+73% 95% CI: 1.05 - 2.84). In comparison with vegan diets, vegetarian diets showed similar trends, but with divergent results between the different cohort studies.

When the data were analyzed by gender, among vegan women, there was no significant risk reduction in incidence of all-cancer (-9%; 95% CI: 0.75 - 1.11), female cancers (-29%; 95% CI: 0.50 - 1.01) and breast cancer (- 17% to − 8%), but data are lacking for other specific sites of cancers. Among vegetarians, similar observations were made for the various types of cancer. However, opposite and non-significant results were shown for breast cancer, ranking from -30% to +14% in the cohort studies analyzed. Dinu et al. reported also in their meta-analysis a small and non-significant reduction of this risk ratio (-6%, 95% CI: 0.84 - 1.06). In addition, vegetarian women experienced a significant increase of cervix cancer (+108%; 95% CI: 1.05 - 4.12).

Among men, vegan diets were also associated with a small and non-significant risk reduction in incidence of all cancers (-19%, 95% CI: 0.57 - 1.17), male cancers (-19%, 95% CI: 0.64 - 1.02). In contrast, prostate cancer incidence was significantly lower (-34%, 95% CI: 0.50 - 0.87) in the Adventist Health Study-2, but that was not the case in the Oxford Vegetarian Study & EPIC-Oxford Cohort (-39%, 95% CI: 0.31 - 1.20). When looking at vegetarian men, conflicting results were observed between the two cohort studies analyz-ing the risk of prostate cancer incidence (-13% and +9%), thus leading to the conclusion that there is only limited evidence for a decreased risk for prostate cancer.

Finally, the differences by diet groups and by gender found for specific causes of cancer incidence merit further investigation.

In conclusion, there is a very small number of available vegan studies, with limited number of cases of cancers in some cohort studies, a large range of follow-ups, the already explained methodological limitations of these observational studies, leading to conflicting results. Further research is still required to prove the potential benefits of vegan diets to lower the risk of cancer incidence, and to demonstrate their advantages over the vegetarian and other plant-diets.

Cancer mortality

A collaborative analysis of data from the first 5 prospective studies, published in 1999 by Key et al. found no significant difference in death rates between vegetarians and non-vegetarians for cancers of the stom-ach, colon-rectum, lung, breast or prostate, but this analysis did not examine overall cancer mortality. However, for vegans data are scarce. The recent publication from Dinu et al. in 2017 is the first systematic review and meta-analysis of observational studies performed to evaluate the association be-tween the vegan and VGT diets and the risk of overall and specific cancer mortality. Otherwise, our review has included the Adventist Health Study-2 and the pooled Oxford Vegetarian Study & EPIC Oxford Study41 in order to assess the consistency of the results between the two populations with different lifestyle habits.

The meta-analysis of Dinu et al. indicates that vegetarian diets including vegan diets were not associated with any significant decrease in the relative risk of mortality from all-cancer (-2%), colon-rectum (-10%), prostate (-10%), lung (-14%) or breast (-6%) in comparison with non-vegetarian diets. Separate analyses for breast cancer mortality exhibited a significant reduction in this risk for the SDA studies (-43%; 95% CI: 0.34 - 0.95), but in contrast, an almost significant increase of + 40% (95% CI: 0.98 - 2.01) for the non-SDA studies. Furthermore, a significant reduction of -41% (95% CI: 0.36 - 0.98) was found in studies with a duration < 14 year, this risk was not significantly increased (+ 38%; 95% CI: 0.82 - 2.30) if the duration was > 14 years. The increased risk of this type of cancer among vegetarians included in the non-SDA studies or in the case of long duration studies remains unexplained. However, these findings require clarification by more specific research before long-term vegetarian diets can be recommended.

In the Adventist Health Study-2, a similar light and non-significant reduced risk of all-cancer mortality was associated with vegan and vegetarian diets when data for men and women were combined. However, divergent results were observed when results were stratified by sex.

Even if the relative risk of overall cancer mortality among vegetarians was the same in the Adventist Health Study-2(-8%; 95% CI: 0.78 - 1.08) and in the Oxford Vegetarian Study & EPIC Oxford Study41 (-9%; 95% CI: 0.80 - 1.03), vegans exhibited conflicting results (-8%; 95% CI: 0.68 - 1.24 versus +10%; 95% CI: 0.85 - 1.42). Moreover, the relative risk of mortality by specific cancers tended to increase in the UK cohort study among ovo-lacto-vegetarians and inversely to decrease in the meta-analysis from Dinu et al. among the vegetarians. The data collected in the available observational studies are not sufficient to explain the dis-crepancies reported here. It must be recognized however that survival in individuals with diagnosed cancer depends on multiple factors, including the treatment modalities not taken into account in the presented studies. These methodological limitations lead to a C-level score of scientific evidence for recommendations. No studies were found investigating the therapeutic impact of vegan or vegetarian diets for cancer survivors.

The scientific evidence available to date is still insufficient to consider whether vegan and vegetarian diets are associated with a significant reduction in risk of mortality by all cancers and mortality by specific cancers reported here; on the contrary Appleby et al. show a non-significant increased mortality risk for breast cancer and other cancers, for pooled vegetarian diets.

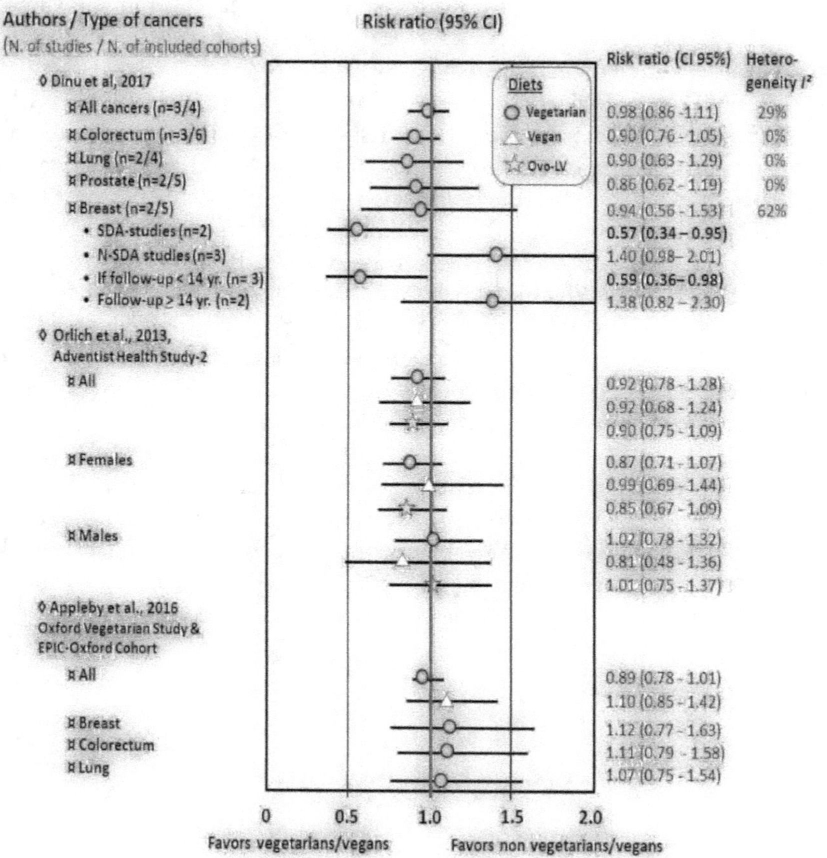

Risk ratio for cancer mortality and specific type of cancers according to the types of vegetarian diets as compared to non-vegetarian diets, Ovo-LV: ovo-lacto-vegetarian

All-cause mortality

Assuming that vegan diets are maintained for the long term, clearly their impact on major health outcomes such as total mortality requests should be indicated. Our review has identified only two prospective cohort studies (Orlich, Appeleby) and the meta-analysis from Dinu et al. already mentioned above.

Vegans exhibited a non-significant reduced risk of total mortality (-12%; 95% CI: 0.75 - 1.02) as compared to non-vegetarian diets in the meta-analysis from Dinu et al.

A similar result was observed for vegan participants in the Adventist Health Study-2 (-15% CI: 0.73 - 1.01), however with differences between men (- 28%; 95% CI: 0.56 - 0.92, significant) and women (-3%; 95% CI: 0.78 - 1.20, non-significant)196. These results contrast with those seen among the vegans included in the Oxford Vegetarian Study & EPIC Oxford Study (+11 %; 95% CI: 0.94 - 0.30, non-significant), as compared to regular meat eaters.

For the vegetarians, the meta-analysis from Dinu et al. shows contrasting results between the Adventist and non-Adventist studies, and between the studies with duration < or > 14 years. Once again, as presented in the Adventist Health Study-2, vegan diets appear to have an increased protective effect in men, more than in women.

In a collaborative analysis of five prospective studies published in 1999, Key et al. concluded that there were non-significant differences between vegetarians and non-vegetarians in all-cause mortality of 0.95 (95% CI: (0.82 - 1.11). Stratified by specific diets, a mortality ratio of 1.0 (95% CI: 0.70 - 1.44) was reported for the vegans and of 0.84 (95% CI: 0.74 - 0.96) for ovolacto-vegetarians excluding vegans.

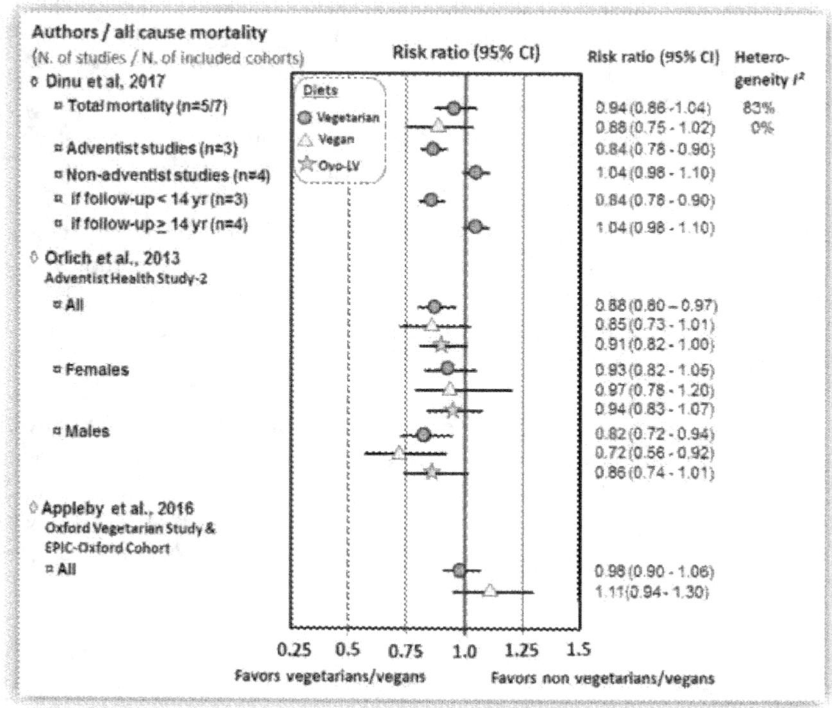

Risk ratio for all-cause mortality according to the types of VGT diets as compared to non VGT diets, ovo-LV: ovo- lacto-vegetarian.

Such heterogeneity of risks remains unclear, based on the available data. Therefore, further research is necessary to determine whether vegan and vegetarian diets could reduce the risk of total mortality in com-parison to non-vegetarian diets, independently of other healthier lifestyle choices.

Due to the small number of studies with sufficient methodological quality and to the limitations of the studies reported here, the scientific evidence available to date is not sufficient to claim that vegan and vegetarian diets are associated with a significant reduction of total mortality. Moreover, these data suggest that vegan diets do not seem to provide advantages over other vegetarian diets. According to the importance of this issue, further research is required to confirm that long-term vegan or vegetarian diets can be associated with a significant reduction of all-cause mortality.

Vegan diets and other diseases

Bone frailty

Some concern has been expressed on the consequences of a long-term vegan diet on bone health, which in general decreases with age. Long-term studies on the impact of a prolonged vegan diet on bone health are not (yet) available. However, possible risk factors could be calcium intake (and its bioavailability) and vitamin D status, as well as changes in the bone mineral density (BMD), already in younger vegans. A plant based diet could however also to contain several bone-protecting constituents such as magnesium, potas-sium, vitamin K, and antioxidant and anti-inflammatory phytonutrients.

BMD is frequently used as indicator of bone health. In a meta-analysis of the BMD of vegetarians in com-parison to omnivores, mainly based on Asian case-control studies and with small number of participants, the authors conclude that vegetarians and especially vegans tend to have a significantly lower BMD but that „the effect size is unlikely to result in a clinically important increase in fracture risk".

A major limitation of this meta-analysis of 9 case-control studies is however that age and duration of the vegan diet were not taken into account.

Lower and not significant BMD (including T and Z-scores) measurements were also observed by Knurick et al.213 in 28 young vegans (average age 33.9 +/-8.6) as compared with 27 omnivores (average age 27.2 +/-6.7). Then vegan group had significantly lower potential renal acid load (PRAL). The authors also stress that these results cannot be extended to bone health with the ageing. Contradictory data on the BMD of vegans vs. vegetarians and omnivores could be explained by an incomplete assessment of various dietary factors, besides calcium and protein intake, e.g. the variability in the nutritional acid load, depending on the fruit and vegetable intake. Conflicting statements show that the evidence of a protective effect of a diet with a low PRAL on bone health is not proved.

Appleby et al. performed an analysis of the data from the EPIC-Oxford cohort study, comparing fracture rates between 1'026 vegan participants and 19'289 meat-eaters (during an average of 5.2 years of follow-up)62. The results show that vegans, when compared to meat eaters, exhibit a non-significant increased incidence rate ratio (IRR) for all bone fractures, with +15% (95% CI: 0.89 - 1.49) for both sexes combined, as well as for men +20% (95% CI: 0.73 – 1.98) and as for women +5% (95% CI: 0.76 – 1.44), when adjusted for confounding factors.

The incidence rate ratio of a bone fracture was neutral (RR 1.00 (95% CI: 0.69-1.44), when comparing meat-eaters to a sub-group of vegans (n= 569), consuming at least 525 mg calcium / day (this also applies to other vegetarian diets). These authors conclude that "the higher fracture risk among vegans appeared to be a consequence of their considerably lower mean calcium intake".

In the same study results for vegetarians (consuming dairy products) showed slightly lower, but non-signif-icant, IRRs when compared to meat-eaters: +0.0% (95% CI: 0.89 - 1.13) for both sexes combined, as well as for men +1% (95% CI: 0.77 - 1.33) and as for women -2% (CI 95% CI: 0.85-1.12).85

Interestingly, Tucker et al in their review have assessed the risks of low nutrients intakes for bone health and have given the description of possible sources of such critical nutrients for vegans.

Irritable bowel syndrome

Irritable bowel syndrome (IBS) is a common functional gastrointestinal disorder (FGID) worldwide. In Swit-zerland, IBS affects 5 to 20% of the adult population, with female predominance. The pathophysiology of IBS is not completely understood, but several abnormalities appear to contribute to its pathogenesis, includ-ing dysregulation of the brain-gut axis, gut dysmotility, visceral hypersensitivity, low-grade mucosal inflam-mation, increased intestinal permeability and altered microbiota. Its aetiology is multifactorial and at least two thirds of patients with IBS relate their GI symptoms to the ingestion of specific foods. Recent attention has been focused on FODMAPs (Fermentable Oligo-, Di-, and Monosaccharides, and Polyols, or oligo-, di-and mono-saccharides and fermentable polyols) which may tend to promote the emergence or exacerbation of IBS in persons sensitive to this functional colopathy. On the other hand, fibers supplementation has recently been advocated to improve the symptoms of IBS, but conflicting results were reported. Typical dietary recommendations in IBS are focused mainly on what foods to avoid and such advices in-cludes a reduce intake of insoluble fibres. As vegan and vegetarian diets are characterised by in-creased dietary intakes of non-soluble fibres as well as plant-based foods rich in FODMAPs, some particular features related to vegan and vegetarian diets could worsen or improve IBS symptoms.

The available scientific data on this topic remain scarce, with only 3 recent publications comparing vegetarian diets to omnivorous diets.

In the cross-sectional data analysis of the Australian Longitudinal Study on Women's Health 9'113 women (aged 22–27 years), Baines et al.225 reported significant higher rates of constipation or other bowel problems among vegetarians (22.7 %) than non-vegetarians (29.1 %, p < 0.001).

A cross-sectional study performed by Ghoshal et al. among 2'774 subjects in a rural Indian population found that participants with a predominantly vegetarian diet were more at risk for IBS (adjusted OR = 10.77, 95% CI: 1.49 to 77.89) than those with a non-vegetarian diet. However, due to the different methodological limitations of this study, namely the very large 95% CI, and the lifestyle habits of the participants, such results cannot be generalised to other populations.

The third paper by Buscail et al. is more appropriate for an assessment of the association between IBS and vegetarian diets in our country. The NutriNet-Santé study is a web-based prospective observational co-hort started in France in 2009 and still ongoing with subjects enrolled at the time of the study. Among them, 41 subjects provided information on vegan and vegetarian diets before answering the FGID questionnaire. Participants were mainly women (78.0%) and the mean age was 49.8 +/-14.3 years. Overall 2'264 (5.4%) subjects reported an IBS, with a higher prevalence in women compared to men (5.6% vs 4.8%, P = 0.03). Anyone who reported to be following a vegetarian/vegan diet at least once was consid-ered as a vegetarian (n = 1'031). Participants who declared at least 3 times that they followed a vegetar-ian/vegan diet (either at baseline or throughout the yearly follow-up questionnaires in NutriNet-Santé) were considered as stable vegetarians (n = 131).

The multivariate analyses by logistic regression models adjusted for age, educational level, total energy intake, income level, smoking status, BMI, physical activity and gender has shown a non-significant trend of higher risk of IBS (odds ratio = 1.24, 95% CI: 0.95 to 1.62) among the vegans/vegetarians. This risk was significantly higher among the small number of stable vegan/vegetarians (odd ratio = 2.66, 95% CI: 1.51 to 4.68). According to the limitations of their cross-sectional NutriNet-Sante cohort, namely the definition of the vegan/vegetarian group and the small number of stable vegetarians, these authors concluded, "this study suggests that a long term vegetarian diet could be associated with IBS. Nevertheless, further studies are needed to confirm these results, and investigate the multiple aspects of the vegetarian diet, possibly related to the IBS".

In summary, in agreement with Buscail et al. further research is required to clarify whether vegan and vegetarian diets are susceptible to positively or negatively influence the emergence and intensity of symp-toms related to IBS. Various web sites contain information to help subjects with IBS who want to start or continue a vegan or vegetarian diet by further restricting it to fulfil low FODMAP requirements, but the effectiveness of this restricted dietary approach has not yet been established.

Fertility disorders

Improper diets and defective nutrition have been linked to a large number of diseases in humans. Emerg-ing evidence, however support lifestyle factors and nutrition as having impact on fertility. Despite the considerable interest focused on vegetarian diets to improve health, the role of vegetarian diets rich in soy foods concerning male fertility remains unclear. The concern lies in the fact that isoflavones in soy foods exert oestrogen-like effects on sperm in vitro and in-vivo, thus in bringing about the possible adverse effects of infertility and feminisation in men who consume soy products. A study from 2008 concerning semen quality in male partners of subfertile couples from an infertility clinic in Boston showed an inverse asso-ciation between soy food intake during the three previous months and sperm concentration this remained significant after accounting for age, abstinence time, body mass index, caffeine and alcohol intake and smoking.

To examine the effect of a life-long vegetarian diet on male fertility, Orzylowska et al. of Loma Linda Adventist University in California carried out this study among members of the Seventh-day Adventist community living in the Loma Linda blue zone, a demographic area known for life longevity. The sperm charac-teristics of ovo-lacto-vegetarians (mean age = 36.2. ± 1.1 years) and vegans (mean age = 40.8 ± 6.9 years) were compared to non-vegetarian controls (mean age = 35.3 ± 0.3 years). Overall, ovo-lacto-vegetarians had a significantly lower sperm concentration (50.7 ± 7.4 million/ml) in comparison to non-veg-etarians (69.6 ± 3.2 million/ml). Furthermore, total motility was lower in the ovo-lacto-vegetarians (33.2 ± 3.8% versus non-vegetarians 58.2 ± 1.0%). Although vegans had a numerically lower concentration (51.0 ± 13.1 million/ml) and lower total sperm motility (51.8 ± 13.4%), these results were not statistically significantly different from non-vegetarians. The authors suggest that phytoestrogens and isoflavones in soy may be exerting a negative effect on sperm quality, but the data need to be carefully interpreted in light of the extremely small number of subjects studied, and effective phytoestrogen intake should be taken into account.

Case reports also exist which support a supplementation of phytoestrogens for promoting fertility in men. Additional studies in which men were randomised to receive low or high doses of isoflavone supplementation to their diets found no significant differences in sperm parameters between the two groups.

It has also been speculated that a lower fertility in general may be related to pesticide exposure, e.g. through fruit and vegetable consumption. A recent study with patients of a fertility clinic (not focused on vegetarian diets) showed that the amounts of pesticide residues in non-organically produced fruits and vegetables were associated with lower total sperm counts and lower percentages of morphologically normal sperm. Specific data linking vegan / vegetarian diets, pesticide residues and fertility were not found.

For women, the scientific literature is very scarce and of low scientific evidence. A 2014 Canadian observa-tional study provided a descriptive profile of self-reported lifestyle habits of young women with infer-tility, the authors found that a high number of women reported past or present eating disorders (27.3%), vegetarian diets (26%, including 2% vegan). On older study by Pedersen et al. studied 41 non-vegetarian and 34 vegetarian premenopausal women, included in two groups that were indistinguishable with respect to height, weight, body mass index, and menarche. The incidence of menstrual irregularity was 4.9% among non-vegetarians and 26.5% among vegetarians (P = 0.009).

Overall, despite the paucity of available data, the results presented here suggest that long-term vegan and vegetarian diets could negatively affect fertility in males and in females. More research is clearly necessary to investigate the impact of a vegan diet and other lifestyle / environmental aspects on fertility. In the mean-time, applying the principle of precaution, counselling on the possible consequences on their fertility should be given to young subjects wishing to adopt or maintain such diets.

Mental diseases and eating disorders

Mental diseases

Mental diseases are a major public health concern, with 27% of the Swiss population concerned. 18.0% of the population have symptoms from moderate (13.4%) to high (4.6%) psychological distress. Depression and anxiety are the most common psychic illnesses, with women being more affected, and younger people more than older people.

During the last decade, increasing knowledge has emerged about the effects of vegan and vegetarian diets on physical health, as seen in the previous chapters. However, little data is available on the associations between vegetarian (vegan included) diets and mental health. On a biological level, nutrition status result-ing from vegan and vegetarian diets may affect brain processes relevant for onset and maintenance of mental disorders.

Besides differences in nutrition status, vegetarians and non-vegetarians differ in a number of psycho-logical and socio-demographic characteristics that may also influence their risk for mental disorders.

To date, no data have been reported on the potential risk of mental diseases related to vegan diets. Con-flicting results, based mainly on cross-sectional studies, do not allow to conclude whether vegetarian diets (vegan diets included) are associated with positive or negative influences on mental health aspects such as mood, emotions, anxiety, depression.

These discrepancies can result mainly from various methodological approaches, size and selection of pop-ulations, nutritional surveys and self-reported mental disorders.

The recent German report by Michalak et al. based on a prospective longitudinal study, can contribute to clarify this relevant clinical issue. Adults aged between 18 and 65 years were recruited between 1998 and 1999 in the German National Health Interview and Examination Survey and its Mental Health Supplement (GHS-MHS). This representative nationwide epidemiological study focused on major somatic and mental disorders, impairments, and healthcare utilization. In addition to physical assessments and com-prehensive questionnaires about health-related behaviors and a nutrition survey, a standardized individual face-to-face diagnostic interview was performed by clinically trained interviewers (psychologists and physi-cians) to detect a broad spectrum of mental disorders.

In the sample, 1.3% (n = 54) of the participants were following exclusively vegetarian diets, 4.5% (n = 190) were on predominantly vegetarian diets, and 94.2% (n=3'872) non-vegetarians. The vegetarian participants were matched with socio-economical similar non-vegetarians (n= 242). Significant socio-economic factors were being age, age, sex, marriage status, community size, education).

A consistent pattern emerged with a gradual increase in prevalence of mental disorders over time, depend-ing on the type of diets. Higher odds ratios for anxiety and unipolar depression were asso-ciated with the degree of adherence to vegetarian diets when compared to the non-vegetarian matched sample. However, for somatoform disorders the extent of odd ratios was similar between the completely and completely / predominantly vegetarian groups.

Importantly, these authors indicate that "no evidence for a causal role of vegetarian diet in the etiology of mental disorders was found. Rather, the results were more consistent with the view that the experience of a mental disorder increases the probability of choosing a vegetarian diet, or that psychological factors influ-ence both the probability of choosing a vegetarian diet and the probability of developing a mental disorder".

Mental disorders	Completely vegetarians	Predominantly vegetarians	Non-vegetarians (total sample)	Non-vegetarians (matched sample)	Comparison completely/ predominantly vegetarians vs. matched non-vegetarians	Comparison completely vegetarians vs. matched non-vegetarians
Time sequencing	(N=54)	(N=190)	(N=3872)	(N=242)	OR (95% CI)	OR (95% CI)
Unipolar Depressive Disorders						
1-month	7.4%	6.8%	6.3%	5.0%	1.44 (0.67 to 3.07)	1.53 (0.48 to 4.95)
12-month	24.1%	14.7%	11.9%	10.3%	**1.75** (1.03 to 2.99)	**2.75** (1.30 to 5.82)
Lifetime	35.2%	25.8%	19.1%	20.7%	1.48 (0.98 to 2.26)	2.09 (1.10 to 3.95)
Anxiety Disorders						
1-month	20.4%	12.6%	10.7%	8.7%	1.76 (0.99 to 3.13)	**2.69** (1.12 to 5.99)
12-month	31.5%	9.5%	17.0%	13.2%	**1.87** (1.15 to 3.01)	**3.02** (1.52 to 5.98)
Lifetime	31.5%	22.1%	18.4%	15.3%	**1.77** (1.12 to 2.79)	**2.55** (1.30 to 4.99)
Somatoform Disorders and Syndromes						
1-month	9.3%	12.1%	7.8%	4.5%	**2.72** (1.32 to 5.60)	2.14 (0.71 to 6.44)
12-month	16.7%	17.9%	11.6%	9.5%	**2.04** (1.19 to .50)	1.90 (0.83 to 4.39)
Lifetime	25.9%	25.8%	16.9%	15.3%	**1.93** (1.23 to 3.03)	1.94 (0.96 to 3.91)

Prevalence rates of mental *disorders*, *by time sequencing*, *in the completely vegetarians*, *predominantly* vegetari-ans, non-vegetarians (total and matched) samples

The relatively simple one-item measure of vegetarian diet and the small number of completely vegetarians presents a limitation to this cohort study. The socio-economic matching suggests that other risk factors are involved in the development of mental disorders.

In summary, despite the rarity of the scientific knowledge and the complexity of the mental disorders, the recent available data suggest that vegetarian diets could be associated with a higher risk of mental disorders. Due to the burden of mental disorders, well-designed intervention studies need to be performed to investigate possible causal patterns between vegan / vegetarian diets and mental disorders. These studies should take into account confounding psychological factors, which could affect both the choice of a vege-tarian diet and the incidence of mental disorders, and possible nutrient deficiencies (e.g. vitamin B12, iron, iodine, long-chain PUFAs).

Eating disorders

Veganism shares some common aspects with restrained eating behaviours, thus leading to the question whether veganism can be associated with extreme forms of restrained eating, in particular eating disorders such as anorexia nervosa, bulimia, or binge eating. Research in this field is scarce, due to the low prevalence of people following a vegan diet and possible selection biases when recruiting participants for this type of study. The few recent studies are in general cross-sectional and are based on either assessing the prevalence of eating disorders in vegetarian / vegan subjects, or on assessing the dietary preferences of subjects diagnosed with eating disorders. All studies are performed with a limited number of participants and using different methodologies, thus making comparisons difficult. The limitations of these studies make it impossible to imply any causality. The studies are difficult to compare, due to the heterogeneity in the approaches, not only in the classification of the diets (self-reported, or based on specific questionnaires), but also in the questionnaire batteries used to determine eating disorders.

The largest study with vegans was performed by Heiss et al. with a "Eating Disorder Examination" on vegans and omnivores (2 groups, n=358 vegans, n=220 omnivores, comparable in demographics, BMI, physical activity, smoking and drinking habits). The researchers observed a significantly lower risk for a pathological eating disorder in vegans. Timko et al. also observed more eating disorders in semi-vegetarians, rather than vegans. This issue of restrained eating in semi-vegetarians was also discussed by Forestell et al. These authors emphasize that correct classifications of diet, and of motivations (in particular the drive for thinness) are essential when investigating this topic.

Other studies, in particular those of Bardone-Cone et al., show that there was an association between eating disorders and vegetarianism (vegans were not specifically identified) in their sample. They also identified a weight-related reason for choosing a vegetarian diet. Their results give some weight to the hypothesis mentioned in most articles, that vegetarianism / veganism might be chosen as socially acceptable ways to mask an eating pathology.

Any positive association between vegan diets and eating disorders would thus need more precise analysis; including detailed characterisation of the diets, data on dietary beliefs and eating habits, clear recruitment criteria and a sufficient number of participants. A longitudinal study would permit access to possible causation patterns, as the existing data are more oriented towards investigating whether a pre-existing eating disorder could lead to a vegan lifestyle; few data were found on investigating whether a vegan diet could lead to further dietary restrictions and with time to an eating disorder. In particular Robinson-O'Brien et al. observed that former adolescent vegans "may be at increased risk for extreme unhealthful weight-control behaviours".

A second group of studies in the field of mental health and veganism focused on the effect of diet on mood and stress. The mainly cross-sectional studies vary in the methodological approach and the studied popu-lations and are therefore not comparable results are therefore not conclusive. An overview of some studies is provided by Beezhold et al.

Ethical considerations from the pediatricians

A discussion on the far-reaching risks and benefits of an exclusion diet such as a vegan diet should include medical and ethical considerations, particularly so when children are involved. Within a culturally heteroge-neous society, there is a wide variation in adopted lifestyles and associated diets. In industrialized western countries parents can choose almost any particular lifestyle for their family as long as the rights of others are not infringed. Parents respectively caregivers have the constitutional right to foster their child according to their own preferences. As autonomous person, they have the right to adopt a particular diet for them-selves. If this diet is provided as the sole source of nourishment for the child, the long-term consequences for the dependent child should however be taken into account. Children have little choice in accepting or refusing the food that they are being offered. Consequently, their rights need to be protected by specific laws such as those formulated in the UN-Convention on the Rights of the Child.

Every child should ideally be fed according to accepted guidelines and age specific requirements. The indi-vidual likes and dislikes of the child for certain foods should be respected as far as the age specific minimal or maximal allowances for the different food components are met and are feasible within the means of a particular family. For the adolescent from the age of about 12 years until full legal maturity is reached the preference for a specific diet should be respected as long as the minor is not insisting on a diet, which in the opinion of the caregiver is clearly not appropriate. It remains difficult to generalize when a decision-making-competence for choosing a particular diet is reached. The adoption of a particular diet usually fol-lows a multitude of reasons including emotional and idiosyncratic motives.

In the case of distinct food intolerance as in celiac disease or lactose intolerance or in the case of a child, suffering under anorexia nervosa medical guidelines should be followed. The use of coercion to accept a particular diet can only be accepted if the vital interests of a child at risk cannot be met otherwise as is the case for certain metabolic diseases.

A situation of child abuse should be considered if the caregiver, despite knowing better, enforces a diet upon the child, which according to mainstream opinion is deficient in essential nutrients.

Following a diet which has a proven detrimental effect on future health aspects, due to a too high concen-tration of certain food components such as fats or calories has been discussed in term of parental neglect. Any intervention by the State in such a case has so far been difficult to justify as there are no clearly defined thresholds above which one can speak of potentially irreversible harm when following a specific diet and due to the high regard for the autonomy of parents and the psychological well-being of the child as part of an interfered interfamily relationship.

A difficulty can arise when conflicting opinions about the pros and cons of a particular diet coexist at a particular point in time. From an ethical point of view, the autonomy of the parents has to be brought in line with the right of a particular child for an "open future" who knows that its interests will in the last resort be protected by State authorities.

Different health associations state that well-balanced and planned vegetarian and vegan diets are compatible with a healthy upbringing at all stages of fetal, infant, child and adolescent growth. As there are no reliable studies on the long-term advantages and disadvantages of a vegan diet in early life, we do not recommend an animal product-exclusive vegan diet in the preschool period. The strain of offering an age appropriate diet with the right amount of micro- and macronutrients and the necessity of repeated laboratory examinations to continuously adapt the diet have to be balanced by a hypothetical gain in health quality and the respect for specific belief systems. As the child becomes increasingly more competent to make decisions for his/her own life and the organ systems have become well established, a vegan diet could, based on present knowledge, be followed at a later age to benefit from the positive health effects that have already been described for adults following a vegetarian or vegan life style. If a vegan diet is chosen for an infant and child, we highly recommend that the diet will be accompanied by an advisory nutrition expert until a firm knowledge of possible dangers to a healthy development has been established.

The environmental arguments of Vegan speech

Purpose Of The Analysis

This chapter analyzes the arguments put forward by The Vegan Society (United Kingdom) and the Vegan Society (France) regarding the environmental benefits of the vegan lifestyle in two areas: land occupation and greenhouse gas. It tries to determine, on the basis of the available literature, to what extent these arguments correspond to the state of the science, if any controversies are related to it and whether they deserve to be nuanced or, on the contrary, affirmed more firmly.

Land occupation and deforestation

The speech of the vegan associations

According to the Vegan Society, the vegan diet would require three times less farmland than the conventional Western diet. It would therefore be beneficial in terms of food security, because the availability of land is "one of the main constraints on mass food production". Indeed, the planet would not be able to feed a growing human population, estimated at 9 billion in 2050, based on the omnivorous diet. This is especially true as climate change will put pressure on the availability and quality of agricultural land. The Vegan Society concludes with this: "Quite simply, we do not have enough land to feed a growing population with a diet based on animal products"

The reason is that cattle "consume much more protein, water and calories than they produce". Indeed, most of the ingested proteins would be used for the biological functions of animals.

In addition, the Vegan Society reports that livestock feed crops contribute significantly to deforestation and habitat loss. It states that in Brazil, 2.8 million hectares are used to grow soybeans for European cattle and that according to the World Bank, the share of responsibility of livestock in the destruction of the Amazon rainforest can rise up to 91%. The French Vegan Society also focuses on the impact of livestock in terms of deforestation. It indicates that 60% of deforestation is due to the expansion of agriculture, with converted land mostly serving cattle grazing a phenomenon it calls "forest hamburgerization".

Comparison with literature

Land Surfaces Devoted To Livestock Farming

Livestock is the sector of activity that consumes the most land resources. According to FAO estimates, it uses more than 3,900 million terrestrial hectares on a planet that has about 13,0004 hectares of which 5,000 are agrosystems. This is 30% of the land area and almost 80% of the world's agricultural land dedicated to it. It is mainly pasture that is concerned: pastures occupy about a quarter of the land area, or 3,500 million hectares. The rest consists of 4 Ice-free land.

Animal feed crops, which occupy one third of the cultivated area, ie 470 million hectares.

Taken from a 1997 study, indicates that pasture area has increased six-fold since 1800, with a marked acceleration from 1850. The growing areas have also expanded markedly, and among them, animal feed crops have grown from a very small area to one third of the cultivated area.

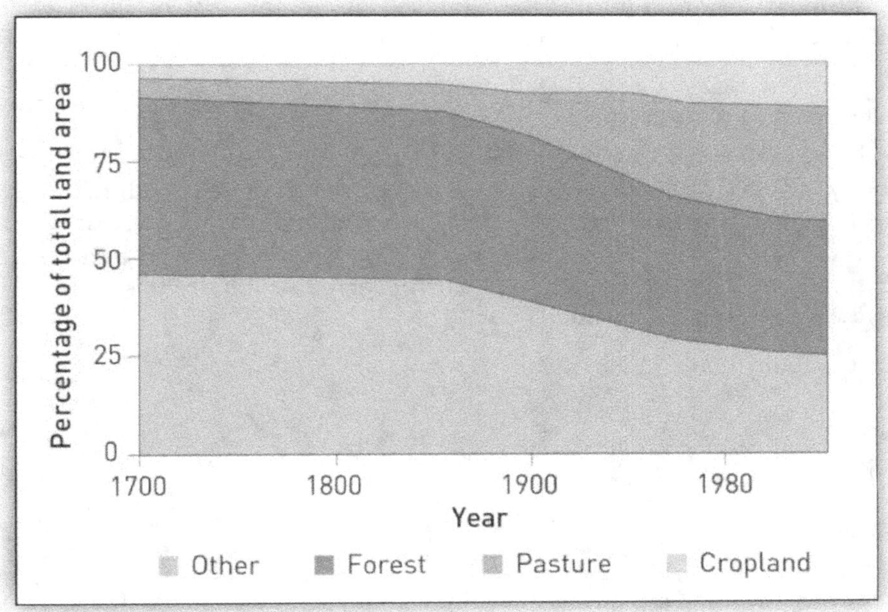

Global areas of forest, pastures and crops from 1700 to 1995
Source: Goldewijk and Battjes, 1997, cited by Steinfeld et al., 2006.

The growth of the land area used for livestock has not been proportional to the increase in production. Indeed, the intensification of production methods has allowed to produce more with less land.

Even if FAO figures are to be taken with caution, in particular because of an imprecise definition of the notion of pastures which can lead to overestimate their surface because it includes ungrazed natural grasslands (Roudart, 2010), they show considerable footprint of the livestock sector.

To these figures could be added the land used for aquaculture, namely those in which aquaculture ponds are located, as well as crop areas for the production of aquaculture feed. In particular, FAO estimated that in 2009, this sector consumed 7 million tonnes of soybeans (out of a total production of 222 million tonnes) to feed on species such as carp and tilapia (Tacon et al., 2011).. Although this element may seem weak or negligible at the moment, it is intended to increase in parallel with aquaculture production. This is the definition of "permanent pastures and pastures" according to FAO.

If animal husbandry and, more generally, the consumption of animal products occupy as much land, would the adoption of a vegan diet be capable of appreciably reducing the footprint of human nutrition, as indicated by the vegan associations? This question will be examined below. But first of all, to what extent does livestock contribute to deforestation?

Livestock and deforestation

While deforestation was intense in the temperate zones until the end of the 19th century, it is mainly in the tropics that it is occurring at present, with the forest growing in temperate and relatively stable in boreal and subtropical areas. Over the period 2000-2010, tropical countries lost on average 7 million hectares of forest per year. Even though the rate of deforestation in this region is decreasing, it is still at an alarming level.

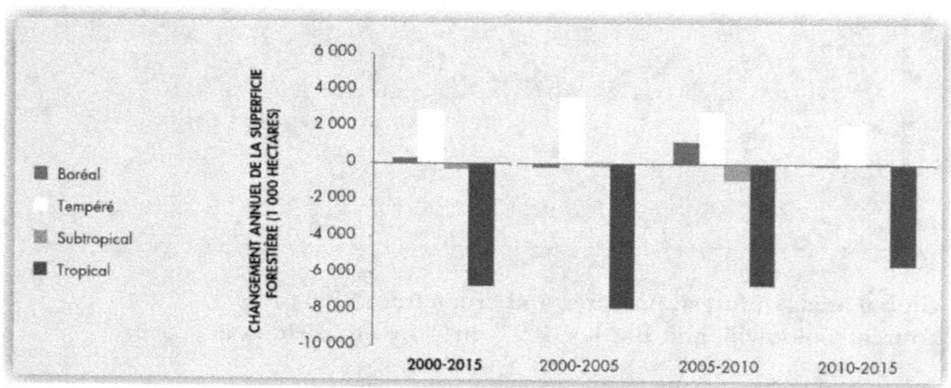

Net change in forest area between 2000 and 2015 by climate zone

The direct causes of deforestation due to human activity are of four types: expansion of agriculture, expansion of infrastructure, expansion of urban areas, and mining. As the vegan associations rightly point out, it is the expansion of agriculture that is the main cause of deforestation. Between 2000 and 2010, she was responsible for about three-quarters (73%) of the phenomenon worldwide, of which 40% was linked to large-scale commercial agriculture and 33% to subsistence farming.

Thus, during this period, while tropical countries lost 7 million hectares of forest per year, they were gaining 6 million hectares of fields and pastures. It should be noted that the figure of 73% is higher than the figure of 60% quoted by the French Vegan Society. In Latin America, it would even reach 90%. Other causes of deforestation (infrastructure, urban areas, mining) are of minor importance and each contribute up to one-tenth of deforestation.

Direct causes of deforestation	Share of deforestation attributable to this cause
Large scale commercial agriculture	40%
Small scale local subsistence agriculture	33%
Infrastructure Expansion	10%
Expansion of urban areas	10%
Mineral extraction	7%

D
irect causes of global deforestation over the period 2000-2010

Regional differences are important with regard to the type of agriculture that causes deforestation: large-scale, export-oriented commercial farming (notably cattle, soybean and palm oil) is considered deforestation (70%) in Latin America, especially in the Amazon region. In Africa and Asia, this type of agriculture accounts for only about one-third of deforestation, equal to or less than that of local subsistence agriculture.

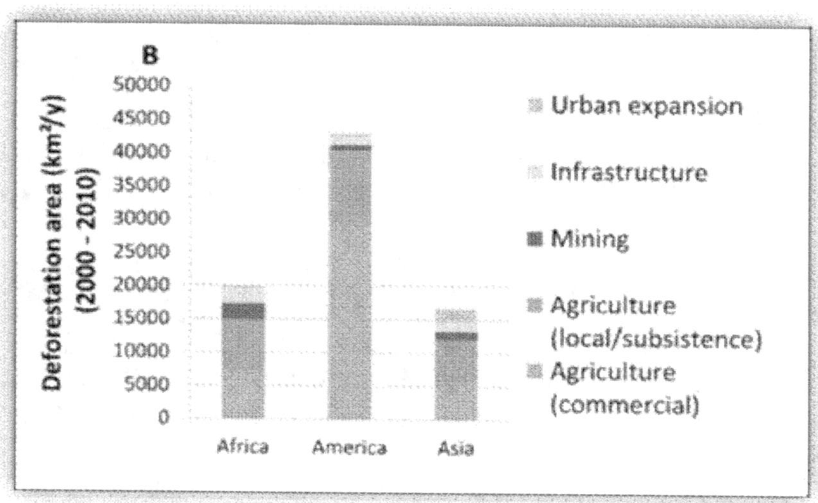

Dir ect causes of deforestation in Africa, America and Asia over the period 2000-2010

What is the specific part of breeding in this process? Several studies have shown that much of the conversion of forest areas to agriculture is linked to cattle rearing, especially in South America.In 2004, the World Bank estimated that livestock   farming.

A large scale of free-range cattle covered nearly 75% of the total deforested areas in the Brazilian Amazon. In 2006, FAO provided a similar estimate that deforestation in the Amazon was mainly due to conversion to pastures (up to 70%) and to feed crops. The latter are mainly soybean crops. Between 1995 and 2005, the size of soybean crops in the Brazilian Amazon doubled to 21 million hectares.

More recently, De Sy et al. (2015) estimated, using satellite remote sensing data, that 71% of the 58 million deforested hectares in Latin America between 1990 and 2005 had been converted to pasture, and 14% to commercial crop areas. In Brazil, 80% of the deforested areas have been converted to pastures over this period. We find here the phenomenon of "hamburgerisation of forests" denounced by the Vegan Society.

In addition, while deforestation has generally slowed down, deforestation in South America has increased between 1990-2000 and 2000-2005, from 3.6 to 4.5 million hectares per year. The development of large cattle farms is identified as one of the main factors of acceleration.

The 91% cited by the Vegan Society (under the terms "Animal agriculture is responsible for up to 91% of Amazon destruction") comes from the World Bank study cited above. It does not concern the total share of the Amazon rainforest lost due to livestock, but the proportion of Brazilian Amazon deforested between 1970 and 1995 that has been converted into free-ranging cattle ranches. Cited out of context, this figure is likely to be confusing.

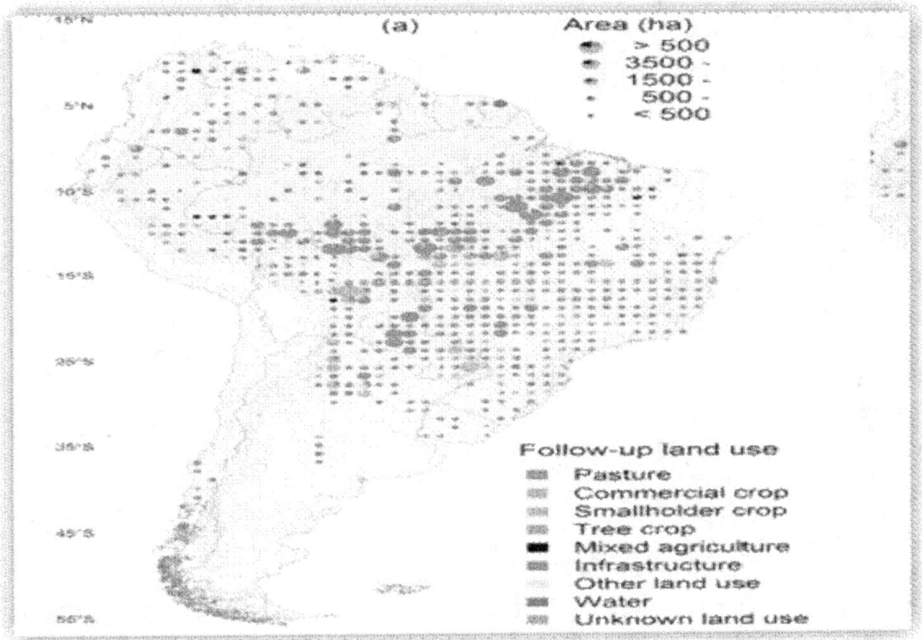

Extent and causes of deforestation in South America between 1990 and 2005

It can be concluded that the arguments put forward by the vegan societies with regard to deforestation are largely corroborated by the literature. The figures quoted must sometimes be adjusted or qualified: some, like the figure of 60% concerning the share of responsibility of agriculture in deforestation, are below the reality, which can be explained by the difficulty of communicating on a phenomenon in constant evolution. Some are cited out of context and are likely to be confusing; this is the case of the expression "up to 91%" which would need to be explained.

Agricultural land availability and food security

The question of the availability of agricultural land to cope with the world's demand for food given the growth of the population and the evolution of food preferences has been the subject of many reflections and publications. The question is whether, as the British economist Malthus theorized, humanity will be faced with a limit in this area because of the growing scarcity of land resources.

In 2006, FAO estimated that land demand from the livestock sector would increase, peak, and then decline due to two conflicting trends: increased production to meet demand, and intensification which reduces the demand for land.

What are the latest estimates available? In their most recent medium-term outlook for global agriculture, which covers the period 2016-2025, the OECD and FAO estimate that by 2025 "the additional food demand will be met through productivity gains, the areas cultivated and the numbers of animals do not change much. Thus, 80% of the additional demand could be satisfied thanks to the increase in agricultural yields. Indeed, many countries have low agricultural yields, particularly in sub-Saharan Africa, and their improvement is likely to greatly increase the world's food supply. The remaining 20% could be covered by an increase in cultivated area. These would increase by 42 million hectares (+ 4%), with the largest increases occurring in Brazil and Argentina.

This expansion of crops would not be entirely linked to the consumption of animal products; only a part of the additional cultivated areas would be dedicated to livestock feed For the longer term, by 2050, projections are very heterogeneous. The results of published studies range from a reduction of 100 million hectares of cultivated area to an increase of 300 million hectares, and even 1,000 Millions of hectares. Uncertainty arises from differences in the structure of the models used, but also from a series of factors related to assumptions about demographic, technological, macroeconomic, climate and public policy developments, including changes in demand. biofuels that can compete with food production. One element that will strongly influence land consumption is the development model that will be chosen for additional agricultural production (extensive model, large land user, or intensive model, which requires investment).

FAO, for its part, estimated that cultivated areas would increase by 70 million hectares by 2050, mainly in sub-Saharan Africa and Latin America. This is a constant public policy estimate based on the 2008 UN population projections, which is lower than current projections (9.1 billion people in 2050 versus 9.7 billion according to the latest projections).

If the cultivated areas are to grow, do we have enough arable land on the planet yet to be cultivated to support this expansion? The answer may seem positive: in 2010, Roudart showed that vast expanses of uncultivated land were available around the world to develop rainfed agriculture. In total, without encroaching on protected areas or forests and considering only the most suitable cropland, more than 500 million hectares would remain available. The areas richest in arable land are South America and sub-Saharan Africa. It is only in Asia and the Middle East that no extension of the crops could be envisaged, the cultivable lands being already used in full. Roudart (2010) concluded that "rainfed land (without the need for irrigation) is not a scarce resource in the world and many regions, limiting agricultural production and food consumption."

Thanks to advances in tools for inventorying land resources and modeling their evolution, estimates are gradually being refined. Thus, in 2012, FAO published higher estimates: 1,400 million hectares would be available globally to expand rainfed crops on good quality land, without encroaching on forests or areas. protected areas and infrastructure areas (Alexandratos and Bruinsma 2012). This represents twenty times the additional area that FAO deems necessary by 2050 to meet world food demand.

The extension potential highlighted and the medium-term projections of OECD and FAO seem to relativize the claims of the Vegan Society and the Vegan Society that "we do not have enough land to feed a growing population. with a diet based on animal products ". The review of the literature shows that there is no scientific consensus on this.

However, the finding of sufficient availability of arable land to meet the future demand for food deserves to be qualified and calls for a number of remarks. First, some authors point out that satellite database reviews - which are the source of the estimates above - may give an inaccurate picture of reality because the information they provide is unclear. In addition, the notion of arable land is a theoretical notion based on the possibility of growing a series of crops in an abstract way. This does not mean that these cultures meet the needs in the region. This can lead to overestimation.

On the other hand, uncultivated land is not necessarily without use. For example, in the estimates quoted above, the extension of cultivated land would be done partly on areas of permanent pastures and pastures. It should be examined to what extent this would include areas actually grazed, as this could result in a "land-use conflict between crops and pastures". Such a conflict of use would be less in areas where pasture areas are not suitable for cultivation. Roudart points to the need for further studies in this area.

The importance of regional disparities must also be emphasized. In fact, the 1,400 million hectares of arable land indicated by FAO as available are in a small number of countries, the other countries having no scope for extension. Although international trade in food is likely to play a growing role, regional or local tensions can not be ruled out. Similarly, the 70 million hectares needed by 2050 according to FAO are the result of an increase of 132 million hectares in some countries, mainly in Latin America and sub-Saharan Africa, and a decrease in 63 million in others, mainly in developed countries. This shows that thinking on a global scale is not the most relevant. As noted by FAO, considering the issue of global food security "is largely meaningless".

In addition, the physical availability of land resources is not the only parameter to be taken into account in assessing the capacity of arable land to play a role in food security. Indeed, this does not only depend on the resources available but also on the way they are used. However, in order to be cultivated, many lands require significant investments, for example in terms of infrastructure, as well as an adequate legal regime for access to land. There can be no assurance that these conditions are met.

The problem of land degradation, which according to the FAO, affects 25% of the world's land, and could be a limiting factor in agricultural production, should also be borne in mind.

Finally, the effects of an extension of agricultural areas on biodiversity and ecosystem services should be examined since some newly cultivated lands would replace natural habitats, especially grassy and wooded areas.

As for the argument of the vegan societies that climate change will put more constraints on the availability of arable land at the global level, it is also nuanced. In fact, it is expected that large areas that are not cultivable in areas that are too cold at the present time can be cultivated at the extremes of both hemispheres and in mountainous regions. On the other hand, in hot regions, the effect on land availability would be negative. These are the regions that are home to the most vulnerable populations and will experience the greatest increase in food needs in the coming decades. Climate change is therefore likely to exacerbate situations of vulnerability. In general, it is considered that the Global warming may negatively affect agricultural production in many parts of the world.
In conclusion, it can be said that the argument that agricultural land will soon be lacking does not seem to be corroborated by the most recent estimates. However, the actual cultivation of additional areas would not be without obstacles and could have negative consequences in terms of biodiversity. At the global level, the availability of arable land is subject to a series of uncertainties linked in particular to changes in demand for biofuels, the consequences of land degradation and the repercussions of global warming.

Impact of dietary change

The feed conversion rate

When animals are raised for human consumption, some of the food they eat is not used to produce food for human consumption (meat, milk or eggs) but is used to make their internal metabolism work, to build inedible tissue and to produce droppings. This phenomenon is reflected by the feed conversion rate, which is the ratio of the amount of food ingested to the amount of animal product obtained at the end of the production process. It measures the efficiency with which the animal transforms food into tissues. The amounts of animal product can be expressed in different ways: by weight, kilocalories or proteins. To calculate the animal product weight, we can consider the total weight of the carcass or only the weight of the edible tissues (which leads to a more unfavorable rate).

The FAO estimated in 1992 that in the case of livestock fed with cereals, each kilocalorie of meat produced requires on average 7 kilocalories of food, which makes animals "poor energy converters". This feed conversion rate varies widely according to the species considered: according to the FAO, in 1992, it varied from 3 for poultry to 16 for cattle. This rate also varies according to the production system considered, and in particular the composition of the food. He has seen great improvements over time. Thus, chicken conversion rates expressed in weight improved by 15% between 1960 and 1995, and those of eggs were improved by 30% during the same period.

Directly consuming the crop product rather than using it to feed the livestock therefore allows efficiency gains, as pointed out by the vegan associations, and therefore land savings. The FAO puts it this way: "The production of animal protein, especially when it depends on the production of other specific crops, is less efficient than the production of vegetable proteins".

However, this reasoning is valid only when the animals fed are with crops that could be used to feed the human population, for example corn or barley. When ruminants are fed on forage from marginal lands that are not suitable for food crops, animal production converts forage into food-grade protein, which in turn generates a net gain in kilocalories for food. Similarly, some farm animals convert products unfit for human consumption, including crop residues (eg corn cane, straw), by-products of the food industry such as cakes, bran, bagasse beet molasses or pulp, or household food waste. In these three cases, abstaining from animal products does not directly save arable land.

In 2002, one-third of the world's cereals were used to feed livestock. This represents 670 million tonnes, equivalent to 211 million hectares of arable land. Cereals are used mainly to feed monogastric species such as pigs and poultry, these species can not digest fodder. It is in intensive livestock systems that the proportion of animal feed from crops is the largest. In 2005, Naylor et al. estimated that this type of farming accounted for 40% of world pork production and three quarters of world poultry production. In the case of ruminants, cereals are generally used as supplements, except in intensive systems such as cattle feedlots or intensive dairy farms where they can form the major part of the diet.

The argument used by vegan associations about the inefficiency of animal production in terms of ingested protein is therefore corroborated by the literature for a large part of the farming systems, particularly the intensive rearing of pigs, poultry and poultry. ruminants in which concentrated cereal-based foods constitute the bulk of the diet. For other types of livestock farming where feed is mixed, consisting of both cereals and fodder, by-products or waste, this statement must be put into perspective. When animals are fed mainly on fodder, this statement is inappropriate. According to the FAO, cattle raised on pasture account for 27% of world beef production

Cassidy et al. attempted to determine how many humans could be fed with the current volume of crops for animal feed. By analyzing the area of arable land dedicated in the year 2000 to the 41 most cultivated species in the world, which are responsible for 91% of plant calories produced worldwide (ie 9.46 x 10 15 calories per year) and FAO's statistics on the use of these crops in different countries (for human food, feed, biofuel or other non-food uses), they deduce that dedicated crops Livestock feed accounts for about one-quarter (24%) of global plant production expressed in weight, over one-third (36%) of this production expressed in calories and more than half (53%) of this production expressed in terms of proteins. The higher proportions of calories and protein are explained by the fact that corn, soybean and oilseeds, which are the basis of animal feed, have a high relative caloric and protein content (Cassidy et al. 2013).

These figures mask important disparities between countries: India, a largely vegetarian country that mainly cultivates rice and wheat, devotes only a small part of the product of its crops to livestock (6% of calories and 18% of calories). % of vegetable protein cultivated), while the United States, the main corn producers, devotes most of its plant production (67% of calories and 80% of protein).

The authors then calculated the share of vegetable calories 6 lost to the human food system by the effect of livestock feed conversion process. They use for this purpose the feed conversion rates (expressed in weight of feed against live weight of the animal) of different cattle species established by the American administration, which they correct to exclude the inedible parts of slaughtered animals, and then convert to calories. They derive indices of dietary conversion efficiency of calories, expressed in percentages, which are relatively low, especially for beef 7, ofwhich 40% of the live weight is considered inedible. Thus, while the conversion rate of beef (expressed as weight of food against live weight) is 12.7, this rate calculated with respect to the edible parts of the animal increases to 21.7, which is more unfavorable.

All species combined, the authors estimate that the process of food conversion causes average losses of 89% of calories from livestock crops. Since these account for 36% of the world's vegetable calories, 32% of the calories from global crops are lost during the conversion process. This figure corresponds to 3.03 x 10 15 calories per year. If these calories were added to those currently used for human consumption, by deducting the crops used for biofuels and other non-food uses (9% of plant calories produced), this would represent a 54% increase in the world's available calories for cooking. human nutrition. Taking into account that the average caloric intake of a human being is 2,700 calories per day, or 985,500 calories per year, this corresponds to the food intake of 3 billion people.

Does this mean that 3 billion more people could be fed on current crops if the choice was made to no longer feed them to livestock? The answer must be nuanced. Indeed, the study has a number of limitations: it excludes life stages of ruminants during which they receive only forage; it does not take into account certain species of ruminants (sheep, goats) that feed exclusively on fodder;and above all, it only considers systems for rearing mixed or above-ground cattle; it does not include cattle raised in pastures. However, as we have seen, these allow a net gain of calories for the food system if they are fed on land unsuitable for cultivation.

Terrestrial footprint of foodstuffs

Other methodologies have been used to estimate the impact of food consumption patterns on land use. Thus, some authors have attempted to define the average land requirements of different foodstuffs. Gerbens-Leenes et al. (2002) defined the specific needs of twenty types of food consumed in the Netherlands, including meat (beef and pork), dairy products (milk, cheese), fruits and vegetables. The land footprint of domestic crops is determined by dividing the total crops of each crop by the areas dedicated to it on the national territory. That of imported crops is based on the volume of imports and average yields of each crop in the country of origin published by FAO. To determine the footprint of animal products, the authors consider the land requirements for fodder and food derived from crops (cereals and legumes) that are fed to animals; By-products and waste from the agri-food industry are not taken into account because their land requirements are fully accounted for for the main food product, excluding by-products or waste that are produced at the same time. When several products are generated by a production system (for example, beef and cow's milk), the land footprint is broken down according to the energy content of each product.

They show that meat (from 8.9 to 20.9) and cheese (10.2) consume much more land than cereals (1.6 for flour), fruit (0.5) and vegetables (0.3). The important difference between beef (20.9) and pork (8.9) stems from the fact that pigs have a higher feed conversion rate than cattle and that they are fed more by-products. the agri-food industry (47% of their average energy intake compared with only 27% for cattle).

It must be kept in mind, however, that these results simplify a complex reality. Caution is warranted in their interpretation as land requirements for food production depend on many parameters, including the rearing system and average yields of crops in the area. In addition, the concept of square meter.

Agricultural land is a fuzzy notion because one hectare of unsuitable pastures is not equivalent to one hectare of top quality arable land.

Footprint of diets

In an attempt to approach the reality more closely, estimates for complete diets have been made. Peters et al. who undertook this exercise, point out that this is a relatively new field of research and that the methodologies used are quite diverse.

Peters et al. compared the land requirements of eight different diets, 8 including the vegan diet, based on the yields and agricultural practices of the United States. All diets assessed have equivalent nutritional content and

The study by Peters et al. (2016) compared to the total of 10 diets. The other two plans are based on the average consumption of Americans over the period 2006-2008, and are not considered here because of their very specific nature.

Follow the national dietary recommendations. Only the protein source differs, illustrating an increasing transition of different diets to vegetable proteins.

The results of this study show a variability from 1 to 7 of land requirements, the most greedy diet (0.93 hectare per person per year) being the 100% omnivorous and least greedy diet (0.13 hectare per person) and per year, being the vegan diet. This result goes well beyond the number 1 to 3 put forward by the vegan associations.

The study divides productive agricultural land into three categories: grazing land, defined as unsuitable for cultivation, arable land used for perennial cropland, and cultivated cropland. "), Defined as those providing food crops (cereals, fruits and vegetables).

It is interesting to note that cropland needs vary little between different diets: from 0.12 to 0.15 hectare per year per person. The difference is mainly in pasture and arable land used for forage crops - ie land directly related to the consumption of animal products.

In addition, the vegan diet requires less cultivated land than the 100% omnivorous diet (0.13 hectare per year and per person against 0.15 hectare per year per person), even though in the vegan diet the All animal proteins - including those from fishery products, which do not consume land - are replaced by vegetable proteins derived from food crops. This is because in the US production system, part of the livestock feed comes from crops such as cereals, and the need to produce these disappears with the adoption of a vegan diet. The situation would be different with a purely grassland rearing system.

Veganism

Veganism is the practice of abstaining from the use of animal products, particularly in diet, and an associated philosophy that rejects the commodity status of animals. A follower of the diet or the philosophy is known as a vegan (/ˈviːgən/ VEE-gən). Distinctions may be made between several categories of veganism. Dietary vegans (or strict vegetarians) refrain from consuming animal products, not only meat but also eggs, dairy products and other animal-derived substances. The term ethical vegan is often applied to those who not only follow a vegan diet but extend the philosophy into other areas of their lives, and oppose the use of animals for any purpose.

Another term is environmental veganism, which refers to the avoidance of animal products on the premise that the industrial farming of animals is environmentally damaging and unsustainable.

Some reviews have shown that some people who eat vegan diets have less chronic disease, including heart disease, than people who do not follow a restrictive diet. They are regarded as appropriate for all stages of life including during infancy and pregnancy by the American Academy of Nutrition and Dietetics, Dietitians of Canada,and the British Dietetic Association. The German Society for Nutrition does not recommend vegan diets for children or adolescents, or during pregnancy and breastfeeding. Vegan diets tend to be higher in dietary fiber, magnesium, folic acid, vitamin C, vitamin E, iron, and phytochemicals; and lower in dietary energy, saturated fat, cholesterol, long-chain omega-3 fatty acids, vitamin D, calcium, zinc, and vitamin B12. Unbalanced vegan diets may lead to nutritional deficiencies that nullify any beneficial effects and may cause serious health issues. Some of these deficiencies can only be prevented through the choice of fortified foods or the regular intake of dietary supplements. Vitamin B12 supplementation is especially important because its deficiency causes blood disorders and potentially irreversible neurological damage.

Donald Watson coined the term vegan in 1944 when he co-founded the Vegan Society in England. At first he used it to mean "non-dairy vegetarian", but from 1951 the Society defined it as "the doctrine that man should live without exploiting animals". Interest in veganism increased in the 2010s, especially in the latter half. More vegan stores opened and vegan options became increasingly available in supermarkets and restaurants in many countries.

History of vegetarianism

The term "vegetarian" has been in use since around 1839 to refer to what was previously described as a vegetable regimen or diet. Modern dictionaries based on scientific linguistic principles explain its origin as an irregular compound of vegetable and the suffix -arian (in the sense of "supporter, believer" as in humanitarian). The earliest-known written use is attributed to the actress Fanny Kemble around 1839 in Georgia in the United States.

The practice can be traced to Indus Valley Civilization in 3300–1300 BCE in the Indian subcontinent, particularly in northern and western India and in Pakistan.

Early vegetarians included Indian philosophers such as Mahavira and Acharya Kundakunda, the Tamil poet Valluvar, the Indian emperors

Chandragupta Maurya and Ashoka; Greek philosophers such as Empedocles, Theophrastus, Plutarch, Plotinus, and Porphyry; and the Roman poet Ovid and the playwright Seneca the Younger. The Greek sage Pythagoras may have advocated an early form of strict vegetarianism, but his life is so obscure that it is disputed whether he ever advocated any form of vegetarianism at all. He almost certainly prohibited his followers from eating beans and from wearing woolen garments. Eudoxus of Cnidus, a student of Archytas and Plato, writes that "Pythagoras was distinguished by such purity and so avoided killing and killers that he not only abstained from animal foods, but even kept his distance from cooks and hunters". One of the earliest known vegans was the Arab poet al-Ma'arri (c. 973 – c. 1057). Their arguments were based on health, the transmigration of souls, animal welfare, and the view—espoused by Porphyry in De Abstinentia ab Esu Animalium ("On Abstinence from Animal Food", c. 268 – c. 270)—that if humans deserve justice, then so do animals.

Vegetarianism established itself as a significant movement in 19th-century England and the United States. A minority of vegetarians avoided animal food entirely. In 1813, the poet Percy Bysshe Shelley published A Vindication of Natural Diet, advocating "abstinence from animal food and spirituous liquors", and in 1815, William Lambe, a London physician, claimed that his "water and vegetable diet" could cure anything from tuberculosis to acne. Lambe called animal food a "habitual irritation", and argued that "milk eating and flesh-eating are but branches of a common system and they must stand or fall together". Sylvester Graham's meatless Graham diet—mostly fruit, vegetables, water, and bread made at home with stoneground flour—became popular as a health remedy in the 1830s in the United States. Several vegan communities were established around this time. In Massachusetts, Amos Bronson Alcott, father of the novelist Louisa May Alcott, opened the Temple School in 1834 and Fruitlands in 1844, and in England, James Pierrepont Greaves founded the Concordium, a vegan community at Alcott House on Ham Common, in 1838.

Vegetarian Society

In 1843, members of Alcott House created the British and Foreign Society for the Promotion of Humanity and Abstinence from Animal Food, led by Sophia Chichester, a wealthy benefactor of Alcott House. Alcott House also helped to establish the UK Vegetarian Society, which held its first meeting in 1847 in Ramsgate, Kent. The Medical Times and Gazette in London reported in 1884:

There are two kinds of Vegetarians—one an extreme form, the members of which eat no animal food whatever; and a less extreme sect, who do not object to eggs, milk, or fish. The Vegetarian Society ... belongs to the latter more moderate division.

The Vegetarian Messenger, in 1851 discussed alternatives to shoe leather, which suggests the presence of vegans within the membership who rejected animal use entirely, not only in diet. By the 1886 publication of Henry S. Salt's A Plea for Vegetarianism and Other Essays, he asserts that, "It is quite true that most—not all—Food Reformers admit into their diet such animal food as milk, butter, cheese, and eggs..." The first known vegan cookbook, Rupert H. Wheldon's No Animal Food: Two Essays and 100 Recipes, was published in London in 1910. The consumption of milk and eggs became a battleground over the following decades. There were regular discussions about it in the Vegetarian Messenger; it appears from the correspondence pages that many opponents of veganism came from vegetarians.

During a visit to London in 1931, Mahatma Gandhi—who had joined the Vegetarian Society's executive committee when he lived in London from 1888 to 1891—gave a speech to the Society arguing that it ought to promote a meat-free diet as a matter of morality, not health. Lacto-vegetarians acknowledged the ethical consistency of the vegan position but regarded a vegan diet as impracticable and were concerned that it might be an impediment to spreading vegetarianism if vegans found themselves unable to participate in social circles where no non-animal food was available. This became the predominant view of the Vegetarian Society, which in 1935 stated: "The lacto-vegetarians, on the whole, do not defend the practice of consuming the dairy products except on the ground of expediency."

Coining the term Vegan

In August 1944, several members of the Vegetarian Society asked that a section of its newsletter be devoted to non-dairy vegetarianism. When the request was turned down, Donald Watson, secretary of the Leicester branch, set up a new quarterly newsletter in November 1944, priced tuppence. He called it The Vegan News. He chose the word vegan himself, based on "the first three and last two letters of 'vegetarian'" because it marked, in Mr Watson's words, "the beginning and end of vegetarian", but asked his readers if they could think of anything better than vegan to stand for "non-dairy vegetarian". They suggested allvega, neo-vegetarian, dairyban, vitan, benevore, sanivores, and beaumangeur.

The first edition attracted more than 100 letters, including from George Bernard Shaw, who resolved to give up eggs and dairy. The new Vegan Society held its first meeting in early November at the Attic Club, 144 High Holborn, London. Those in attendance were Donald Watson, Elsie B. Shrigley, Fay K. Henderson, Alfred Hy Haffenden, Paul Spencer and Bernard Drake, with Mme Pataleewa (Barbara Moore, a Russian-British engineer) observing. World Vegan Day is held every 1 November to mark the founding of the Society and the month of November is considered by the Society to be World Vegan Month.

The Vegan News changed its name to The Vegan in November 1945, by which time it had 500 subscribers. It published recipes and a "vegan trade list" of animal-free products, such as Colgate toothpaste, Kiwi shoe polish, Dawson & Owen stationery and Gloy glue. Vegan books appeared, including Vegan Recipes by Fay K. Henderson and Aids to a Vegan Diet for Children by Kathleen V. Mayo.

The Vegan Society soon made clear that it rejected the use of animals for any purpose, not only in diet. In 1947, Watson wrote: "The vegan renounces it as superstitious that human life depends upon the exploitation of these creatures whose feelings are much the same as our own ...". From 1948, The Vegan's front page read: "Advocating living without exploitation", and in 1951, the Society published its definition of veganism as "the doctrine that man should live without exploiting animals". In 1956, its vice-president, Leslie Cross, founded the Plantmilk Society; and in 1965, as Plantmilk Ltd and later Plamil Foods, it began production of one of the first widely distributed soy milks in the Western world.

The first vegan society in the United States was founded in 1948 by Catherine Nimmo and Rubin Abramowitz in California, who distributed Watson's newsletter. In 1960, H. Jay Dinshah founded the American Vegan Society (AVS), linking veganism to the concept of ahimsa, "non-harming" in Sanskrit. According to Joanne Stepaniak, the word vegan was first published independently in 1962 by the Oxford Illustrated Dictionary, defined as "a vegetarian who eats no butter, eggs, cheese, or milk".

Increasing interest

Alternative food movements

In the 1960s and 1970s, a vegetarian food movement emerged as part of the counterculture in the United States that focused on concerns about diet, the environment, and a distrust of food producers, leading to increasing interest in organic gardening. One of the most influential vegetarian books of that time was Frances Moore Lappé's 1971 text, Diet for a Small Planet. It sold more than three million copies and suggested "getting off the top of the food chain".

The following decades saw research by a group of scientists and doctors in the United States, including physicians Dean Ornish, Caldwell Esselstyn, Neal D. Barnard, John A. McDougall, Michael Greger, and biochemist T. Colin Campbell, who argued that diets based on animal fat and animal protein, such as the Western pattern diet, were detrimental to health. They produced a series of books that recommend vegan or vegetarian diets, including McDougall's The McDougall Plan (1983), John Robbins's Diet for a New America (1987), which associated meat eating with environmental damage, and Dr. Dean Ornish's Program for Reversing Heart Disease (1990). In 2003 two major North American dietitians' associations indicated that well-planned vegan diets were suitable for all life stages. This was followed by the film Earthlings (2005), Campbell's The China Study (2005), Rory Freedman and Kim Barnouin's Skinny Bitch (2005), Jonathan Safran Foer's Eating Animals (2009), and the film Forks over Knives (2011).

In the 1980s, veganism became associated with punk subculture and ideologies, particularly straight edge hardcore punk in the United States; and anarcho-punk in the United Kingdom. This association continues on into the 21st century, as evinced by the prominence of vegan punk events such as Fluff Fest in Europe.

Interest in veganism in the 2010s was reflected in Wikipedia, where vegan pages received more views than vegetarian ones.

The vegan diet became increasingly mainstream in the 2010s, especially in the latter half. The European Parliament defined the meaning of vegan for food labels in 2010, in force as of 2015. Chain restaurants began marking vegan items on their menus and supermarkets improved their selection of vegan processed food.

The global mock-meats market increased by eighteen percent between 2005 and 2010, and in the United States by eight percent between 2012 and 2015, to $553 million a year. The Vegetarian Butcher (De Vegetarische Slager), the first known vegetarian butcher shop, selling mock meats, opened in the Netherlands in 2010, while America's first vegan butcher, the Herbivorous Butcher, opened in Minneapolis in 2016. By 2016, forty-nine percent of Americans were drinking plant milk, although 91 percent still drank dairy milk. In the United Kingdom, the plant milk market increased by 155 percent in two years, from 36 million litres (63 million imperial pints) in 2011 to 92 million (162 million imperial pints) in 2013. The country has seen a 185% increase in new vegan products between 2012 and 2016. In 2011, Europe's first vegan supermarkets appeared in Germany: Vegilicious in Dortmund and Veganz in Berlin.

Veganism has risen in popularity in Hong Kong and China, as well, particularly among millennials. China's vegan market is estimated to rise by more than 17 percent between 2015 and 2020, which is expected to be "the fastest growth rate internationally in that period".This exceeds the projected growth in the second and third fastest-growing vegan markets internationally in the same period, the United Arab Emirates (10.6%) and Australia (9.6%) respectively. In total, as of 2016, the largest share of vegan consumers globally currently reside in Asia Pacific with 9 percent of people following a vegan diet.

Countering the image of self-deprivation projected by vegan straight edges and animal rights activists, veganism was promoted as glamorous; in 2015, the editor of Yahoo! Food declared that it had become "a thing". Celebrities, athletes, and politicians adopted vegan diets—some seriously, some part-time. The idea of the "flexi-vegan" gained currency: New York Times food columnist Mark Bittman, in VB6 (2013), recommended eating vegan food until 6 pm. In 2013, the Oktoberfest in Munich—traditionally a meat-heavy affair— offered vegan dishes for the first time in its 200-year history.

Critics of veganism questioned the evolutionary legitimacy and health effects of a vegan diet, and pointed to longstanding philosophical traditions which held that humans are superior to other animals. Celebrity chef Anthony Bourdain wrote in 2000 that "[v]egetarians, and their Hezbollah-like splinter-faction, the vegans, are a persistent irritant to any chef worth a damn". Several vegetarian writers argued that the restrictions of a vegan lifestyle are impractical, and that vegetarianism is a better goal.

Veganism by country

Vegetarianism by country Demographics

Australia: Australians topped Google's worldwide searches for the word "vegan" between mid-2015 and mid-2016. A Euromonitor International study concluded the market for packaged vegan food in Australia would rise 9.6% per year between 2015 and 2020, making Australia the third-fastest growing vegan market behind China and the United Arab Emirates.

Austria: In 2013, Kurier estimated that 0.5 percent of Austrians practised veganism, and in the capital, Vienna, 0.7 percent.

Belgium: A 2016 iVOX online study found that out of 1000 Dutch-speaking residents of Flanders and Brussels of 18 years and over, 0.3 percent were vegan.

Canada: In 2018, one survey estimated that 2.1 percent of adult Canadians considered themselves as vegans.

Germany: As of 2016, data estimated that people following a vegan diet in Germany varied between 0.1% and 1% of the population (between 81,000 and 810,000 persons).

India: In the 2005–06 National Health Survey, 1.6% of the surveyed population reported never consuming animal products. Veganism was most common in the states of Gujarat (4.9%) and Maharashtra (4.0%).

Israel: Five percent (approx. 300,000) in Israel said they were vegan in 2014, making it the highest per capita vegan population in the world. A 2015 survey by Globes and Israel's Channel 2 News similarly found 5% of Israelis were vegan. Veganism increased among Israeli Arabs. The Israeli army made special provision for vegan soldiers in 2015, which included providing non-leather boots and wool-free berets.

Italy: Between 0.6 and three percent of Italians were reported to be vegan as of 2015.

Netherlands: In 2018, the Dutch Society for Veganism (Nederlandse Vereniging voor Veganisme) estimated there were more than 100,000 Dutch vegans (0.59 percent), based on their membership growth.

Romania: Followers of the Romanian Orthodox Church keep fast during several periods throughout the ecclesiastical calendar amounting to a majority of the year. In the Romanian Orthodox tradition, devotees abstain from eating any animal products during these times. As a result, vegan foods are abundant in stores and restaurants; however, Romanians may not be familiar with a vegan diet as a full-time lifestyle choice.

Sweden: Four percent said they were vegan in a 2014 Demoskop poll.

Switzerland: The Vegan Society Switzerland (Vegane Gesellschaft Schweiz) estimated in 2016 that one percent of the population was vegan.

United Kingdom: In the UK, where the tofu and mock-meats market was worth £786.5 million in 2012, two percent said they were vegan in a 2007 government survey. A 2016 Ipsos MORI study commissioned by the Vegan Society, surveying almost 10,000 people aged 15 or over across England, Scotland, and Wales, found that 1.05 percent were vegan; the Vegan Society estimates that 542,000 in the UK follow a vegan diet. According to a 2018 survey by Comparethemarket.com, the number of people who identify as vegans in the United Kingdom has risen to over 3.5 million, which is approximately seven percent of the population, and environmental concerns were a major factor in this development. However, doubt was cast on this inflated figure by the UK-based Vegan Society, who perform their own regular survey: the Vegan Society themselves found in 2018 that there were 600,000 vegans in Great Britain (1.16%), which is a dramatic increase on previous figures.

United States: Estimates of vegans in the U.S. vary from 2% to 0.5% (Faunalytics, 2014). According to the latter, 70% of those who adopted a vegan diet abandoned it. Top Trends in Prepared Foods 2017, a report by GlobalData, estimated that "6% of US consumers now claim to be vegan, up from just 1% in 2014."

Animal products

Avoidance

Rendering (food processing)

Vegans do not eat beef, pork, poultry, fowl, game, animal seafood, eggs, dairy, or any other animal products. Dietary vegans might use animal products in clothing (as leather, wool, and silk), toiletries, and similar. Ethical veganism extends not only to matters of food but also to the wearing or use of animal products, and rejects the commodification of animals altogether. The British Vegan Society will certify a product only if it is free of animal involvement as far as possible and practical, including animal testing,but "recognises that it is not always possible to make a choice that avoids the use of animals", an issue that was highlighted in 2016 when it became known that the UK's newly-introduced £5 note contained tallow.

An important concern is the case of medications, which are routinely tested on animals to ensure they are effective and safe, and may also contain animal ingredients, such as lactose, gelatine, or stearates. There may be no alternatives to prescribed medication or these alternatives may be unsuitable, less effective, or have more adverse side effects. Experimentation with laboratory animals is also used for evaluating the safety of vaccines, food additives, cosmetics, household products, workplace chemicals, and many other substances.

Philosopher Gary Steiner argues that it is not possible to be entirely vegan, because animal use and products are "deeply and imperceptibly woven into the fabric of human society". Animal products in common use include albumen, allantoin, beeswax, blood, bone char, bone china, carmine, casein, castoreum, cochineal, elastin, emu oil, gelatin, honey, isinglass, keratin, lactic acid, lanolin, lard, rennet, retinol, shellac, squalene, tallow (including sodium tallowate), whey, and yellow grease. Some of these are chemical compounds that can be derived from animal products, plants, or petrochemicals. Allantoin, lactic acid, retinol, and squalene, for example, can be vegan. These products and their origins are not always included in the list of ingredients. Vegetables themselves, even from organic farms, may use animal manure; "vegan" vegetables use plant compost only.

Some vegans will not buy woollen jumpers, silk scarves, leather shoes, bedding that contains goose down or duck feathers, pearl jewellery, seashells, ordinary soap (usually made of animal fat), or cosmetics that contain animal products. They avoid certain vaccines; the flu vaccine, for example, is usually grown in hens' eggs, although an effective alternative, Flublok, is widely available in the United States. Non-vegan items acquired before they became vegan might be donated to charity or used until worn out. Some vegan clothes, in particular leather alternatives, are made of petroleum-based products, which has triggered criticism because of the environmental damage involved in their production.

Eggs and dairy products

Modern methods of factory farming are considered highly unethical by most vegans. The main difference between a vegan and vegetarian diet is that vegans exclude dairy products and eggs. Ethical vegans avoid them on the premise that their production causes animal suffering and premature death. In egg production, most male chicks are culled because they do not lay eggs. To obtain milk from dairy cattle, cows are made pregnant to induce lactation; they are kept lactating for three to seven years, then slaughtered. Female calves can be separated from their mothers within 24 hours of birth, and fed milk replacer to retain the cow's milk for human consumption. Male calves are slaughtered at birth, sent for veal production, or reared for beef.

Honey and silk

Vegan groups disagree about insect products. Neither the Vegan Society nor the American Vegan Society considers honey, silk, and other insect products as suitable for vegans, Insect products can be defined much more widely, as commercial bees are used to pollinate about 100 different food crops.

Pet food

Vegetarian and vegan dog diet, Dog food § Vegetarian and vegan dog food, Cat food § Vegetarian or vegan food, and Cat health § Diet and nutrition

Due to the environmental impact of meat-based pet food and the ethical problems it poses for vegans, some vegans extend their philosophy to include the diets of pets. This is particularly true for domesticated cats and dogs, for which vegan pet food is both available and nutritionally complete, such as Vegepet. However, this practice has been met with caution and criticism, especially toward vegan cat diets due to felids being obligate carnivores. Furthermore, although nutritionally complete vegan pet diets are comparable to meat-based ones for cats and dogs, as of August 2015 many commercial vegan pet food brands do not meet the Association of American Feed Control Officials (AAFCO) regulations for nutritional adequacy.

Vegan diet

Vegan diets are based on grains and other seeds, legumes (particularly beans), fruits, vegetables, edible mushrooms, and nuts.

Soy

Meatless products based on soybeans (tofu), or wheat-based seitan are sources of plant protein, commonly in the form of vegetarian sausage, mince, and veggie burgers.

Soy-based dishes are a staple of vegan diets because soy is a complete protein; i.e. it has all the essential amino acids for humans and can be relied on entirely for protein intake. They are consumed most often in the form of soy milk and tofu (bean curd), which is soy milk mixed with a coagulant. Tofu comes in a variety of textures, depending on water content, from firm, medium firm and extra firm for stews and stir-fries to soft or silken for salad dressings, desserts and shakes. Soy is also eaten in the form of tempeh and textured vegetable protein (TVP); also known as textured soy protein (TSP), the latter is often used in pasta sauces.

Plant milk, cheese, mayonnaise

Nutritional content of cows', soy, and almond milk

Plant milks—such as soy milk, almond milk, grain milks (oat milk, flax milk and rice milk), hemp milk, and coconut milk—are used in place of cows' or goats' milk.[m] Soy milk provides around 7 g (¼oz) of protein per cup (240 mL or 8 fl oz), compared with 8 g (2/7oz) of protein per cup of cow's milk. Almond milk is lower in dietary energy, carbohydrates, and protein. Soy milk should not be used as a replacement for breast milk for babies. Babies who are not breastfed may be fed commercial infant formula, normally based on cows' milk or soy. The latter is known as soy-based infant formula or SBIF.

Butter and margarine can be replaced with alternate vegan products. Vegan cheeses are made from seeds, such as sesame and sunflower; nuts, such as cashew, pine nut, and almond; and soybeans, coconut oil, nutritional yeast, tapioca, and rice, among other ingredients; and can replicate the meltability of dairy cheese. Nutritional yeast is a common substitute for the taste of cheese in vegan recipes. Cheese substitutes can be made at home, including from nuts, such as cashews.

Egg replacements

Tofu can be used as an egg replacement

Egg substitutes

Commercial egg substitutes are available for cooking and baking. The protein in eggs thickens when heated and binds other ingredients together. For pancakes a tablespoon of baking powder can be used instead of eggs. Silken (soft) tofu and mashed potato can also be used. Aquafaba from chickpeas can be used as an egg replacement and whipped like egg whites. Another egg alternative in pastries is banana. Half a banana replaces an egg.

Raw veganism

Raw veganism, combining veganism and raw foodism, excludes all animal products and food cooked above 48 °C (118 °F). A raw vegan diet includes vegetables, fruits, nuts, grain and legume sprouts, seeds, and sea vegetables. There are many variations of the diet, including fruitarianism.

Nutrients

Protein

Protein quality, Pea protein, Protein (nutrient), Protein–energy malnutrition, Rice protein, Soy protein, and Hemp protein

Rice and beans is a common vegan protein combination.

Proteins are composed of amino acids. Vegans obtain all their protein from plants, omnivores usually a third, and ovo-lacto vegetarians half. Sources of plant protein include legumes such as soy beans (consumed as tofu, tempeh, textured vegetable protein, soy milk, and edamame), peas, peanuts, black beans, and chickpeas (the latter often eaten as hummus); grains such as quinoa, brown rice, corn, barley, bulgur, and wheat (the latter eaten as bread and seitan); and nuts and seeds. Combinations that contain high amounts of all the essential amino acids include rice and beans, corn and beans, and hummus and whole wheat pita.

Soy beans and quinoa are known as complete proteins because they each contain all the essential amino acids in amounts that meet or exceed human requirements. Mangels et al. write that consuming the recommended dietary allowance (RDA) of protein 0.8 g/kg (12gr/lb) of body weight in the form of soy will meet the biologic requirement for amino acids. In 2012, the United States Department of Agriculture ruled that soy protein (tofu) may replace meat protein in the National School Lunch Program.

The American Dietetic Association said in 2009 that a variety of plant foods consumed over the course of a day can provide all the essential amino acids for healthy adults, which means that protein combining in the same meal may not be necessary. Mangels et al. write that there is little reason to advise vegans to increase their protein intake; but erring on the side of caution, they recommend a 25 percent increase over the RDA for adults, to 1g/kg (15gr/lb) of body weight.

Vitamin B12

Vitamin B12 deficiency, Vitamin B12 § Supplements, and Food fortification Tahini miso soup with brown rice, turnips, squash, radishes and nori (an edible seaweed). Nori has been cited as a plant source of B12, but the Academy of Nutrition and Dietetics established in 2016 that is not an adequate source of this vitamin. Vegans need to consume regularly fortified foods or supplements containing B12.

Vitamin B12 is a bacterial product needed for cell division, the formation and maturation of red blood cells, the synthesis of DNA, and normal nerve function. A deficiency may cause megaloblastic anaemia and neurological damage, and, if untreated, may lead to death. The high content of folacin in vegetarian diets may mask the hematological symptoms of vitamin B12 deficiency, so it may go undetected until neurological signs in the late stages are evident, which can be irreversible, such as neuropsychiatric abnormalities, neuropathy, dementia and, occasionally, atrophy of optic nerves. Vegans sometimes fail to obtain enough B12 from their diet because among non-fortified foods, only those of animal origin contain sufficient amounts. The best source is ruminant food. Vegetarians are also at risk, as are older people and those with certain medical conditions. A 2013 study found that "vegetarians develop B12 depletion or deficiency regardless of demographic characteristics, place of residency, age, or type of vegetarian diet. Vegans should take preventive measures to ensure adequate intake of this vitamin, including regular consumption of supplements containing B12."

B12 is produced in nature only by certain bacteria and archaea; it is not made by any animal, fungus, or plant. It is synthesized by some gut bacteria in humans and other animals, but humans cannot absorb the B12 made in their guts, as it is made in the colon which is too far from the small intestine, where absorption of B12 occurs. Ruminants, such as cows and sheep, absorb B12 produced by bacteria in their guts.

Animals store vitamin B12 in liver and muscle and some pass the vitamin into their eggs and milk; meat, liver, eggs and milk are therefore sources of B12.

It has been suggested that nori (an edible seaweed), tempeh (a fermented soybean food), and nutritional yeast may be sources of vitamin B12. In 2016, the Academy of Nutrition and Dietetics established that nori, fermented foods (such as tempeh), spirulina, chlorella algae, and unfortified nutritional yeast are not adequate sources of vitamin B12 and that vegans need to consume regularly fortified foods or supplements containing B12. Otherwise, vitamin B12 deficiency may develop, as has been demonstrated in case studies of vegan infants, children, and adults.

Vitamin B12 is mostly manufactured by industrial fermentation of various kinds of bacteria, which make forms of cyanocobalamin, which are further processed to generate the ingredient included in supplements and fortified foods. The Pseudomonas denitrificans strain was most commonly used as of 2017. It is grown in a medium containing sucrose, yeast extract, and several metallic salts. To increase vitamin production, it is supplemented with sugar beet molasses, or, less frequently, with choline. Certain brands of B12 supplements are vegan.

CALCIUM

Vegan cheeses
Calcium is needed to maintain bone health and for several metabolic functions, including muscle function, vascular contraction and vasodilation, nerve transmission, intracellular signalling, and hormonal secretion. Ninety-nine percent of the body's calcium is stored in the bones and teeth.

High-calcium foods may include fortified plant milk or fortified tofu. Plant sources include broccoli, turnip, bok choy, collards, and kale; the bioavailability of calcium in spinach is poor. Vegans should make sure they consume enough vitamin D, which is needed for calcium absorption.

A 2007 report based on the Oxford cohort of the European Prospective Investigation into Cancer and Nutrition, which began in 1993, suggested that vegans have an increased risk of bone fractures over meat eaters and vegetarians, likely because of lower dietary calcium intake. The study found that vegans consuming at least 525 mg (8gr) of calcium daily have a risk of fractures similar to that of other groups. A 2009 study found the bone mineral density (BMD) of vegans was 94 percent that of omnivores, but deemed the difference clinically insignificant.

VITAMIN D

Vitamin D deficiency, Rickets, and Hypervitaminosis D. Vitamin D (calciferol) is needed for several functions, including calcium absorption, enabling mineralization of bone, and bone growth. Without it bones can become thin and brittle; together with calcium it offers protection against osteoporosis. Vitamin D is produced in the body when ultraviolet rays from the sun hit the skin; outdoor exposure is needed because UVB radiation does not penetrate glass. It is present in salmon, tuna, mackerel and cod liver oil, with small amounts in cheese, egg yolks, and beef liver, and in some mushrooms.

Most vegan diets contain little or no vitamin D without fortified food. People with little sun exposure may need supplements. The extent to which sun exposure is sufficient depends on the season, time of day, cloud and smog cover, skin melanin content, and whether sunscreen is worn. According to the National Institutes of Health, most people can obtain and store sufficient

vitamin D from sunlight in the spring, summer, and fall, even in the far north. They report that some researchers recommend 5–30 minutes of sun exposure without sunscreen between 10 am and 3 pm, at least twice a week. Tanning beds emitting 2–6% UVB radiation have a similar effect, though tanning is inadvisable.

Vitamin D comes in two forms. Cholecalciferol (vitamin D3) is synthesized in the skin after exposure to the sun or consumed from food, usually from animal sources. Ergocalciferol (vitamin D2) is derived from ergosterol from UV-exposed mushrooms or yeast and is suitable for vegans. When produced industrially as supplements, vitamin D3 is typically derived from lanolin in sheep's wool. However, both provitamins and vitamins D2 and D3 have been discovered in Cladina spp. (especially Cladina rangiferina) and these edible lichen are harvested in the wild for producing vegan vitamin D3. Conflicting studies have suggested that the two forms of vitamin D may or may not be bioequivalent. According to researchers from the Institute of Medicine, the differences between vitamins D2 and D3 do not affect metabolism, both function as prohormones, and when activated exhibit identical responses in the body.

Iron

Human iron metabolism, Iron supplement, and Iron deficiency

Oatmeal with blueberries, toasted almonds and almond milk; one packet of instant oatmeal contains 8.2 mg (1/8gr) of iron.

In some cases iron and the zinc status of vegans may also be of concern because of the limited bioavailability of these minerals. There are concerns about the bioavailability of iron from plant foods, assumed by some researchers to be 5–15 percent compared to 18 percent from a nonvegetarian diet. Iron-deficiency anemia is found as often in nonvegetarians as in vegetarians, though studies have shown vegetarians' iron stores to be lower.

Mangels et al. write that, because of the lower bioavailability of iron from plant sources, the Food and Nutrition Board of the National Academy of Sciences established a separate RDA for vegetarians and vegans of 14 mg (¼gr) for vegetarian men and postmenopausal women, and 33 mg (½gr) for premenopausal women not using oral contraceptives. Supplements should be used with caution after consulting a physician, because iron can accumulate in the body and cause damage to organs. This is particularly true of anyone with hemochromatosis, a relatively common condition that can remain undiagnosed.

High-iron vegan foods include soybeans, blackstrap molasses, black beans, lentils, chickpeas, spinach, tempeh, tofu, and lima beans. Iron absorption can be enhanced by eating a source of vitamin C at the same time, such as half a cup of cauliflower or five fluid ounces of orange juice. Coffee and some herbal teas can inhibit iron absorption, as can spices that contain tannins such as turmeric, coriander, chiles, and tamarind.

OMEGA-3 FATTY ACIDS, IODINE

Essential fatty acid interactions, Iodine in biology, and Iodine deficiency. Alpha-linolenic acid (ALA), an omega-3 fatty acid, is found in walnuts, seeds, and vegetable oils, such as canola and flaxseed oil. EPA and DHA, the other primary omega-3 fatty acids, are found only in animal products and algae. Iodine supplementation may be necessary for vegans in countries where salt is not typically iodized, where it is iodized at low levels, or where, as in Britain and Ireland, dairy products are relied upon for iodine delivery because of low levels in the soil. Iodine can be obtained from most vegan multivitamins or regular consumption of seaweeds, such as kelp.

Health research

Vegan nutrition
Supermarket freezer stocked with packaged food
Vegan products in a supermarket (Oceanside, California, 2014)

As of 2014, few studies were rigorous in their comparison of omnivore, vegetarian, and vegan diets, making it difficult to discern whether health benefits attributed to veganism might also apply to vegetarian diets or diets that include moderate meat intake.

In preliminary clinical research, vegan diets lowered the risk of type 2 diabetes, high blood pressure, obesity, and ischemic heart disease. A 2016 systematic review from observational studies of vegetarians showed reduced body mass index, total cholesterol, LDL cholesterol, and glucose levels, possibly indicating lower risk of ischemic heart disease and cancer, but having no effect on mortality, cardiovascular diseases, cerebrovascular diseases, and mortality from cancer.

Eliminating all animal products may increase the risk of deficiencies of vitamins B12 and D, calcium, and omega-3 fatty acids. Vitamin B12 deficiency occurs in up to 80% of vegans that do not supplement with vitamin B12. Vegans might be at risk of low bone mineral density without supplements. Lack of B12 inhibits normal function of the nervous system.

Many vegans overestimate the health benefits of a vegan diet, which has resulted in victim blaming when vegans fall ill.

Professional and Goverment associations

The American Academy of Nutrition and Dietetics and Diettians of Canada state that properly planned vegan diets are appropriate for all life stages, including pregnancy and lactation. They indicate that vegetarian diets may be more common among adolescents with eating disorders, but that its adoption may serve to camouflage a disorder rather than cause one. The Australian National Health and Medical Research Council similarly recognizes a well-planned vegan diet as viable for any age. The British National Health Service's Eatwell Plate allows for an entirely plant-based diet, as does the United States Department of Agriculture's (USDA) MyPlate. The USDA allows tofu to replace meat in the National School Lunch Program. The German Society for Nutrition does not recommend a vegan diet for babies, children and adolescents, or for women pregnant or breastfeeding.

Pregnancy, infants and children

Nutrition and pregnancy

The Academy of Nutrition and Dietetics and Dietitians of Canada consider well-planned vegetarian and vegan diets "appropriate for individuals during all stages of the lifecycle, including pregnancy, lactation, infancy, childhood, and adolescence, and for athletes". The German Society for Nutrition cautioned against a vegan diet for pregnant women, babies, and children as of 2011. The position of the Canadian Pediatric Society is that "well-planned vegetarian and vegan diets with appropriate attention to specific nutrient components can provide a healthy alternative lifestyle at all stages of fetal, infant, child and adolescent growth. Attention should be given to nutrient intake, particularly protein, vitamins B12 and D, essential fatty acids, iron, zinc, and calcium.

According to a 2015 systematic review, there is little evidence available about vegetarian and vegan diets during pregnancy, and a lack of randomized studies meant that the effects of diet could not be distinguished from confounding factors. It concluded: "Within these limits, vegan-vegetarian diets may be considered safe in pregnancy, provided that attention is paid to vitamin and trace element requirements." A daily source of vitamin B12 is important for pregnant and lactating vegans, as is vitamin D if there are concerns about low sun exposure. A different review found that pregnant vegetarians consumed less zinc than pregnant non-vegetarians, with both groups' intake below recommended levels; however, the review found no significant difference between groups in actual zinc levels in bodily tissues, nor any effect on gestation period or birth weight.

Researchers have reported cases of vitamin B12 deficiency in lactating vegetarian mothers that were linked to deficiencies and neurological disorders in their children. A doctor or registered dietitian should be consulted about taking supplements during pregnancy.

Vegan diets have attracted negative attention from the media because of cases of nutritional deficiencies that have come to the attention of the courts, including the death of a baby in New Zealand in 2002 due to hypocobalaminemia, i.e. vitamin B12 deficiency.

Personal items

Testing cosmetics on animals

Vegan soap made from olive oil; soap is usually made from tallow (animal fat).

Vegans replace personal care products and household cleaners containing animal products with products that are vegan, such as vegan dental floss made of bamboo fiber. Animal ingredients are ubiquitous because they are relatively inexpensive. After animals are slaughtered for meat, the leftovers are put

through a rendering process and some of that material, particularly the fat, is used in toiletries.

Common animal-derived ingredients include: tallow in soap; collagen-derived glycerine, which used as a lubricant and humectant in many haircare products, moisturizers, shaving foams, soaps and toothpastes; lanolin from sheep's wool is often found in lip balm and moisturizers; stearic acid is a common ingredient in face creams, shaving foam and shampoos, (as with glycerine, it can be plant-based, but is usually animal-derived); Lactic acid, an alpha-hydroxy acid derived from animal milk, is used in moisturizers; allantoin— from the comfrey plant or cows' urine —is found in shampoos, moisturizers and toothpaste; and carmine from scale insects, such as the female cochineal, is used in food and cosmetics to produce red and pink shades;

Animal Ingredients A to Z (2004) and Veganissimo A to Z (2013) list which ingredients might be animal-derived. The British Vegan Society's sunflower logo and PETA's bunny logo mean the product is certified vegan, which includes no animal testing. The Leaping Bunny logo signals no animal testing, but it might not be vegan. The Vegan Society criteria for vegan certification are that the product contain no animal products, and that neither the finished item nor its ingredients have been tested on animals by, or on behalf of, the manufacturer or by anyone over whom the manufacturer has control. Its website contains a list of certified products, as does Australia's Choose Cruelty Free (CCF).

Beauty Without Cruelty, founded as a charity in 1959, was one of the earliest manufacturers and certifiers of animal-free personal care products. Several international companies produce animal-free products, including clothes, shoes, fashion items, and candles.

Vegans avoid clothing that incorporates silk, wool (including lambswool, shearling, cashmere, angora, mohair, and a number of other fine wools), fur, feathers, pearls, animal-derived dyes, leather, snakeskin, and any other kind of skin or animal product. Most leather clothing is made from cow skins. Vegans regard the purchase of leather, particularly from cows, as financial support for the meat industry. Vegans may wear clothing items and accessories made of non-animal-derived materials such as hemp, linen, cotton, canvas, polyester, artificial leather (pleather), rubber, and vinyl. Leather alternatives can come from materials such as cork, piña (from pineapples), and mushroom leather.

Philosophy

Ethical veganism

Carnism and Ethics of eating meat

Pigs, as well as chicken and cattle, are often denied freedom of movement and other basic rights.

Ethical veganism is based on opposition to speciesism, the assignment of value to individuals on the basis of species membership alone. Divisions within animal rights theory include the utilitarian, protectionist approach, which pursues improved conditions for animals. It also pertains to the rights-based abolitionism, which seeks to end human ownership of non-humans. Abolitionists argue that protectionism serves only to make the public feel that animal use can be morally unproblematic (the "happy meat" position).

Law professor Gary Francione, an abolitionist, argues that all sentient beings should have the right not to be treated as property, and that adopting veganism must be the baseline for anyone who believes that non-humans have intrinsic moral value. Philosopher Tom Regan, also a rights theorist, argues that animals possess value as "subjects-of-a-life", because they have beliefs, desires, memory and the ability to initiate action in pursuit of goals. The right of subjects-of-a-life not to be harmed can be overridden by other moral principles, but Regan argues that pleasure, convenience and the economic interests of farmers are not weighty enough. Philosopher Peter Singer, a protectionist and utilitarian, argues that there is no moral or logical justification for failing to count animal suffering as a consequence when making decisions, and that killing animals should be rejected unless necessary for survival. Despite this, he writes that "ethical thinking can be sensitive to circumstances", and that he is "not too concerned about trivial infractions".

An argument proposed by Bruce Friedrich, also a protectionist, holds that strict adherence to veganism harms animals, because it focuses on personal purity, rather than encouraging people to give up whatever animal products they can. For Francione, this is similar to arguing that, because human-rights abuses can never be eliminated, we should not defend human rights in situations we control. By failing to ask a server whether something contains animal products, we reinforce that the moral rights of animals are a matter of convenience, he argues. He concludes from this that the protectionist position fails on its own consequentialist terms.

Philosopher Val Plumwood maintained that ethical veganism is "subtly human-centred", an example of what she called "human/nature dualism" because it views humanity as separate from the rest of nature. Ethical vegans want to admit non-humans into the category that deserves special protection, rather than recognize the "ecological embeddedness" of all. Plumwood wrote that animal food may be an "unnecessary evil" from the perspective of the consumer who "draws on the whole planet for nutritional needs"—and she strongly opposed factory farming—but for anyone relying on a much smaller ecosystem, it is very difficult or impossible to be vegan.

Bioethicist Ben Mepham, in his review of Francione and Garner's book The Animal Rights Debate: Abolition or Regulation?, concludes that "if the aim of ethics is to choose the right, or best, course of action in specific circumstances 'all things considered', it is arguable that adherence to such an absolutist agenda is simplistic and open to serious self-contradictions. Or, as Farlie puts it, with characteristic panache: 'to conclude that veganism is the "only ethical response" is to take a big leap into a very muddy pond'." He cites as examples the adverse effects on animal wildlife derived from the agricultural practices necessary to sustain most vegan diets and the ethical contradiction of favoring the welfare of domesticated animals but not that of wild animals; the imbalance between the resources that are used to promote the welfare of animals as opposed to those destined to alleviate the suffering of the approximately one billion human beings who undergo malnutrition, abuse, and exploitation; the focus on attitudes and conditions in western developed countries, leaving out the rights and interests of societies whose economy, culture and, in some cases, survival rely on a symbiotic relationship with animals.

David Pearce, a transhumanist philosopher, has argued that humanity has a "hedonistic imperative" to not merely avoid cruelty to animals or abolish the ownership of non-human animals, but also to redesign the global ecosystem such that wild animal suffering ceases to exist. In the pursuit of abolishing suffering itself, Pearce promotes predation elimination among animals and the "cross-species global analogue of the welfare state". Fertility regulation could maintain herbivore populations at sustainable levels, "a more civilised and compassionate policy option than famine, predation, and disease". The increasing number of vegans and vegetarians in the transhumanism movement has been attributed in part to Pearce's influence.

A growing political philosophy that incorporates veganism as part of its revolutionary praxis is veganarchism, which seeks "total abolition" or "total liberation" for all animals, including humans. Veganarchists identify the state as unnecessary and harmful to animals, both human and non-human, and advocate for the adoption of a vegan lifestyle within a stateless society. The term was popularized in 1995 with Brian A. Dominick's pamphlet Animal Liberation and Social Revolution, described as "a vegan perspective on anarchism or an anarchist perspective on veganism". Direct action is a common practice among veganarchists (and anarchists generally) with groups like the Animal Liberation Front (ALF) and Revolutionary Cells – Animal Liberation Brigade (RCALB) often engaging in such activities, sometimes criminally, to further their goals.

Some extreme sects of vegans also embrace the philosophy of anti-natalism, as they see the two as complementary in terms of "harm reduction" to animals and the environment.

Environmental Veganism

Environmental vegetarianism, Feed conversion ratio, and Vegan organic gardening. Environmental vegans focus on conservation, rejecting the use of animal products on the premise that fishing, hunting, trapping and farming, particularly factory farming, are environmentally unsustainable. In 2010, Paul Watson of the Sea Shepherd Conservation Society called pigs and chicken "major aquatic predators", because livestock eat 40 percent of the fish that are caught. Since 2002, all Sea Shepherd ships have been vegan for environmental reasons. This specific form of veganism focuses its way of living on how to have a sustainable way of life without consuming animals.

According to a 2006 United Nations Food and Agriculture Organization report, Livestock's Long Shadow, 222 million tonnes of meat were produced globally in 1999. The report posits that around 26 percent of the planet's terrestrial surface is devoted to livestock grazing. In the United States ten billion land animals are killed every year for human consumption, and in 2005 48 billion birds were killed globally.

The UN report also concluded that livestock farming (mostly of cows, chickens and pigs) affects the air, land, soil, water, biodiversity and climate change. Livestock consumed 1,174 million tonnes of food in 2002—including 7.6 million tonnes of fishmeal and 670 million tonnes of cereals, one-third of the global cereal harvest—and in 2001 consumed 45 million tonnes of roots and vegetables and 17 million tonnes of pulses. As of 2006, the livestock industry accounted for nine percent of anthropogenic carbon dioxide emissions, 37 percent of methane, 65 percent of nitrous oxide, and 68 percent of ammonia. Livestock waste emitted 30 million tonnes of ammonia a year, which is involved in the production of acid rain. A 2017 study published in the journal Carbon Balance and Management found animal agriculture's global methane emissions are 11% higher than previous estimates based on data from the Intergovernmental Panel on Climate Change. A June 2018 study published in Science asserted that the adoption of plant-based diets in the United States alone could cut greenhouse gas emissions by 61% to 73%, and the global adoption of a vegan diet would reduce the use of agricultural land by 75%.

A 2010 UN report, Assessing the Environmental Impacts of Consumption and Production, argued that animal products "in general require more resources and cause higher emissions than plant-based alternatives". It proposed a move away from animal products to reduce environmental damage. A 2007

Cornell University study concluded that vegetarian diets use the least land per capita, but require higher quality land than is needed to feed animals. A 2015 study published in Science of the Total Environment determined that significant biodiversity loss can be attributed to the growing demand for meat, which is a significant driver of deforestation and habitat destruction, with species-rich habitats being converted to agriculture for livestock production. A 2017 study by the World Wildlife Fund found that 60% of biodiversity loss can be attributed to the vast scale of feed crop cultivation needed to rear tens of billions of farm animals, which puts an enormous strain on natural resources resulting in an extensive loss of lands and species. Livestock make up 60% of the biomass of all mammals on earth, followed by humans (36%) and wild mammals (4%). As for birds, 70% are domesticated, such as poultry, whereas only 30% are wild. In November 2017, 15,364 world scientists signed a warning to humanity calling for, among other things, "promoting dietary shifts towards mostly plant-based foods". According to a July 2018 study in Science, meat consumption is set to increase as the result of human population growth and rising affluence, which will increase greenhouse gas emissions and further reduce biodiversity.

Farmers in the United States could sustain more than twice as many people than they do currently if they abandoned rearing farm animals for human consumption and instead focused on growing plants.

Feminist Veganism

Vegetarian ecofeminism Pioneers

One of the leading activists and scholars of feminist animal rights is Carol J. Adams. Her premier work, The Sexual Politics of Meat: A Feminist-Vegetarian Critical Theory (1990), sparked what was to become a movement in animal rights as she noted the relationship between feminism and meat consumption. Since the release of The Sexual Politics of Meat, Adams has published several other works including essays, books, and keynote addresses. In one of her speeches, "Why feminist-vegan now?"—adapted from her original address at the "Minding Animals" conference in Newcastle, Australia (2009)—Adams states that "the idea that there was a connection between feminism and vegetarianism came to [her] in October 1974", illustrating that the concept of feminist veganism has been around for nearly half a century. Other authors have also paralleled Adams' ideas while expanding on them. Angella Duvnjak states in "Joining the Dots: Some Reflections on Feminist-Vegan Political Practice and Choice" that she was met with opposition to the connection of feminist and veganism ideals, although the connection seemed more than obvious to her and other scholars (2011). Other scholars elaborate on the connections between feminism, such as Carrie Hamilton who makes the connection to sex workers and animal reproductive rights. Many other scholars of feminist vegan philosophy continue to add to the arguments that Adams, Duvnjak, and Hamilton have brought forth.

Animal and human abuse parallels

Some of the main concepts of feminist veganism is that is the connection between the violence and oppression of animals. For example, Marjorie Spiegal compares the consumption or servitude of animals for human gain to slavery. Animals are purchased from a breeder, used for personal gain— either for further breeding or manual labor—and then discarded, most frequently as food. This capitalist use of animals for personal gain has held strong, despite the work of animal rights activists and ecofriendly feminists.

Similar notions that suggest animals—like fish, for example—feel less pain are brought forth today as a justification for animal cruelty. The feminist side of the argument, however, suggests that there is no rationalization for treating animal lives with lesser reverence than human lives, even if the theory that animals are less capable of pain is verifiable.[citation needed]

Another connection between feminism and veganism is the parallel of violence against women or other minority members and the violence against animals. Animal rights activists closely relates animal cruelty to feminist issues. This connection is even further mirrored as animals that are used for breeding practices are compared to human trafficking victims and migrant sex workers. Hamilton points out that violent "rapists sometimes exhibit behavior that seems to be patterned on the mutilation of animals" suggesting there is a trend between the violence towards rape victims and animal cruelty previously exhibited by the rapist.

The violence connection is not limited to sexual acts, however. It is a common fact the prevalence of violence against animals are more defined in those with psychopathic disorders. This mirroring of violence against animals and violence against weaker animals lead the pioneers of feminist veganism to suggest that there is a correspondence between violence against humans and animals, supporting feminist veganism.

Capitalism and feminist veganism

Another way that feminist veganism relates to feminist thoughts is through the capitalist means of the production itself. Carol J. Adams mentions Barbara Noske talking about "meat eating as the ultimate capitalist product, because it takes so much to make the product, it uses up so many resources". The capitalization of resources for meat production is argued to be better used for production of other food products that have a less detrimental impact on the environment.

Symbols

Vegetarian and vegan symbolism

Multiple symbols have been developed to represent veganism. Several are used on consumer packaging, including the Vegan Society trademark and Vegan Action logo, to indicate products without animal-derived ingredients. Various symbols may also be used by members of the vegan community to represent their identity and in the course of animal rights activism,[citation needed] such as a vegan flag.

Vegtarianism

Vegetarianism is a food practice that excludes animal meat consumption. Its broadest definition is egg-lacto-vegetarianism consisting of eating plants, fungi, and animal origin foods (such as honey, eggs, milk and derivatives). This is the classical Western vegetarianism that its practitioners were called "Pythagoras / Pythagoras" until 1847. but excludes eggs (Manu's law also excludes mushroom consumption).

Vegetarianism is practiced for various reasons. Some are vegetarians because of ethics, religion, cultural or health. The adoption of the vegetarian diet can be motivated by other factors: criticism of traceability methods, reproduction and sacrifice, access to food, environmental impacts of production methods and their collection of food. energy and water conservation; or animal exploitation in principle.

Some studies have reported that a variety of disease risks, including those with vegetarian (or almost vegetarian), vegan or vegetarian diets (including cardiovascular disease and insulin-resistant diabetes), are reduced and the risk of general death is reduced. compared to those who regularly consume meat; This risk reduction is more pronounced in men. However, according to previous studies, this health benefit is also observed in non-vegetarians who are concerned about their health and can be associated with more lifestyle than the diet itself.

In general, all dietary applications, including the consumption of other animal products, except animal meat, are called "vegetarianism" and "vegetarian" practitioners. Fish, crustaceans and aquatic crustaceans, or vegetarianism (or lik pestaryanism zaman) vegetarianism, often called (semi-vegetarianism (,have other dietary practices. Occasional meat consumption. On the other hand, vegan excludes all products of animal origin.

The word "vegetarian" is derived from English and appears as an adjective in 1873 and as a name in 1875. The Vegetarian Community, founded in 1847, writes that the Latin vegetus has created the word vegetarian. In the old homo vegetus, it means "healthy, fresh and alive", which is the expression of a human for a healthy body and mind. The Latin term "-ism" refers to the concept of the system. The Oxford English Dictionary states that it was used in Ramsgate after the formation of the Vegetarian Society in 1839, but gave two examples in 1839 and 1842.

Forms

There are several forms of vegetarianism:
Ovo-lacto-vegetarianism, the most common practice in Western countries, includes eggs, dairy products (cheese, butter, yoghurts ...) and honey.

Contains "lactose-vegetarianism" (or "Indian vegetarian") dairy products, but does not cover eggs, including those found in processed products, such as some pasta and many cakes.

In contrast to lactose-vegetarianism, "Ovo vegetarianism" includes eggs and dairy products.

Veganism peynir includes only plants (more minerals or microorganisms such as yeast or bacteria) and excludes any animal product (including eggs, milk, cheese and honey). Veganism includes the other two more restrictive diet patterns:

Fruit production consists of eating only plant materials that can be collected without damaging fruits, nuts, seeds and plants. The principle of this diet is to destroy only the ripe fruit of the trees to eat the plants that can be prevented to a certain extent. Therefore, a fruit grower can eat beans, tomatoes, zucchini, but may refuse to eat tubers and spinach.

Crudicananismo is not about cooking foods over 48 ° C and eating only raw fruits and vegetables, nuts and nuts, grains and pulses seeds, seeds, and oils. plants, herbal seas, aromatic plants and fresh fruits. Juices Raw food eaters eat raw food for health reasons.

Type of vegetarianism	Animal flesh and by-products of slaughtered animals	Milk and derivatives	Eggs and derivatives	Honey and derivatives	Mushrooms, yeasts and derivatives	Plants and derivatives
Lacto-ovo-vegetarianism	Non	Yes	Yes	Yes	Yes	Yes
Lacto vegetarianism	Non	Yes	Non	Yes	Yes	Yes
Ovo-vegetarianism	Non	Non	Yes	Yes	Yes	Yes
Vegetarianism ,veganism	Non	Non	Non	Non	Yes	Yes
Crudi-vegetalism	Non	Non	Non	Non	Yes *but only raw*	Yes *but only raw*

Summary table of types of vegetarianism

Special non-vegetarian diets

The following diets are not vegetarian but close

Calar pezo-vegetarianism ini (or pesterianism içeren), which contains the most known flesh of aquatic animals (fish, crustaceans and molluscs). This diet is applied by the Cathars in the Middle Ages. It is also recommended by Dr. Andrew Weil, MD in his book On Healthy Eating for Optimal Health (Good Nutrition for Optimal Health). This Lenten diet is close to the dietary practices of Catholics on Fridays and every Friday, more traditionally. Although many people accept themselves as vegetarians, the menu includes fish that protects from confusion between pesevtarizm and vegetarianism.

"Flexitarianism" refers to the inclusion of products of animal origin in a vegetarian diet. In the case of people consuming poultry, seafood or fish, we will speak of "semi-vegetarianism".

The "macrobiotic" approach was defined by Georges Ohsawa: a philosophical discipline of food based on the principle of yin and yang. This system consists of ten ways to feed the numbers: -3, -2, -1, 1, 2, 3, 4, 5, 6, 7. Levels -3 to 3 are not vegetarian. No. 4 to 7 vegan is salad, raw vegetables and fruits. A macrobiotic can circulate at all levels and is not necessarily vegetarian or vegan.

Related Apps

"Veganism", in addition to being vegan, also applies to those who refrain from using any animal product (cosmetics tested on skin, wool, fur, wax and animals).

A vegan accepts products that do not belong to a process that is only attracted to an animal: plants, minerals or micro-organisms (not tested on animals). This is actually based on the definition of and vegetarian and in the Hindu world, just before the term iddiddet vegan inden and practicing practically all violence in a short period of time (serving or bringing meat into contact). An animal is considered contrary to ahimsa and therefore contrary to "vegetarianism" as defined in Manu's law, for example - verses 5, 55, verse

The word "vegetarianism" is XIX. It turns out that in the 17th century, this practice was called first "abstinence", then at least in the West "xerofaji" or "plant diet"; According to the so-called artist Claude Augé, until now, vegetarians in Europe have been called "philosophers", that is to say the philosopher Pythagoras or "legumists". Indeed, it is true that the honor of setting the vegetarian diet, called "Pythagorean diet," is attributed to Pythagoras, even though his practices are not known. Pythagoras declares that he defends the return to vegetarianism and refuses to kill animals; Blood shed (golden age), but a few hundred years later, the biographies contradict each other and order him to classify the victims of various animals. Unlike the Indian subcontinent, where the vegetarian, vegetarian and ahimsa doctrine has spread to different communities since prehistory, it is limited to philosophical or religious sects. Moreover, in Europe, a non-vegetarian reaction develops with a philosopher like Aristotle, and there are Stoics who awaken animals that have the right to use animals and to use their flesh and that create a hierarchy between their lives.

In China, the Daoists of the Laozi era defended the vegetation. Under their influence, the banqueting tradition has turned into a vegetarian festival where alcohol has remained one of the main elements of the tradition.

Middle Ages

The collapse of ancient culture Middle Ages at the same time the Christian plays the shell of vegetarianism in the West. Like the heterodox movements, it is still being applied for a reclusive lifestyle. The Cathars (peso vegetarian) or monkhood. The last one to see fasting and vegetarianism as forms of redemption. While meat dishes are regarded as the privilege of upper classes in the Renaissance, they emerge as a philosophical concept based on ethical considerations with personalities like vegetarianism. Thomas More or Erasmus. Leonardo da Vinci, by witnesses of the time as a follower of vegetarianism, but there is no evidence that she is vegetarian: on the contrary, the race charts, which last for the rest of her life, show that she regularly consumes animal products. In xvii pearl century develops scientific vegetarianism with philosophers Isaac Newton, Pierre Gassendi and Francis Bacon Saying that a vegetarian diet is the most suitable diet for humans and that its authors and evangelist are religious vegetarianism Thomas Tryon, One of the first theoreticians of vegetarianism. Researcher Arouna Ouedraogo, a vegetarian discourse xviii pearl centuries of themes (crusades for health, rejection of persecution of animals) "Part of the self-righteous categories of vegetarianism that progeny uses to promote their diets".

Vegeterian diet, For all men, this is the primary logic that motivates the application nonviolent especially with many philosophical trends Indian (Hindu, Sikhs, Jain and Buddhists As part of, ahimsa) and Greeks (predominantly Orphism, Pythagorism and students Empedocles) as well as several Jewish personalities and movements (Essenes for example), Christians and Muslim (in mysticism).

Throughout its history, ethical and non-violent size vegetarianism is supported by many people (and not always, always): Plato, the Theophrastus Apollonius of Tyana, Plutarch, Sicilian philosopher Empedocles, Phoenician philosopher Tire Porphyry, Latin poets Ovid, Virgil, Horace and Latin philosopher Plotinus. In India contain philosophers Mahavira (and all Tîrthankar Show) Patanjali (and all yogis), Adi Shankara, Madhva, Chaitanya

Mahaprabhu, Swaminarayan, AC Bhaktivedanta Swami Prabhupada, Ciddu Krishnamurti, Siddhartha Gautama (Buddha), Indian Emperor Ashoka, Indian mathematician Srinivasa Ramanujan, Indian poet and philosopher Guru Nanak, Hindu philosopher Jambheshwar Bhagavan, Indian poet Rabindranath Tagore, Tamil poet Tiruvalluv is, Mahatma Gandhi (clearly with a trend vegetalis Poet Aziz, adopted between 1911-1917, but abandoned for health reasons) Grave and dancer and Indian politician Rukmini Devi Arundale.

A few sources show Adolf Hitler, He was a vegetarian from the 1930s. . However, other sources indicate otherwise: Charles Patterson Adolf Hitler never gave up his favorite meat dishes, and Victor Klemperer, He recalls that the German dictator ordered, and that the Jews destroyed all their pets. Gang leader and serial killer Charles Manson, Pol Pot and Volkert Van der Graaf also vegetarians.

In Iranian, they are Iranian prophets Zarathustra, slashing and author Sadegh Hedayat. In United States of America, physicist Albert Einstein, Dexter Scott King, philosopher Amos Bronson Alcott, doctor John Harvey Kellogg and Polish-American writer Isaac Bashevis Singer. In United Kingdom , English poet Percy Shelley, English poet Sir byron, Irish writer George Bernard Shaw and British feminist Anna Kingsford. In France philosopher Voltaire, poet and politician Alphonse de Lamartine, author Jacques-Henri Bernardin de Saint-Pierre, geographer and anarchist Élisée Reclus, philosopher and Alsatian doctor Albert Schweitzer, Belgian writer Marguerite Yourcenar, actress Brigitte Bardot, journalist Aymerik Caron.

And all over the world, Iraqi Muslim mystic Rabia al Adawiyya, Chinese Emperor Wudi, Japanese Emperor the term, Indian King Kumārapāl to Italian artist Léonard de Vinci, Flemish artists Pierre Paul Rubens Burmese politician Aung San Suu Kyi, Arab poet Abu-l-Ala el-Maari (vegan) Russian writer Leo Tolstoy, British philosopher David Hartley, Czech writer Franz Kafka Israeli writer Samuel Joseph Agnon, Belgian writer Maurice Maeterlinck.

Currently, such as celebrities Paul McCartney with Olivia Harrison , Yoko Ono, Sheryl Crow, Jeff Beck, Bryan Adams, and For Moby form Meat Free Monday, "Meatless Monday "Increase awareness of the impact of meat consumption on the ecosystem:" consume less meat for a better world", As well as Lutan Fyah and Matthieu Ricard devoted vegetarian. Global meat consumption rises almost sevenfold between 1950 and 2012 revitalizing vegetarianism in industrialized countries for ethical reasons and ecologic.

Global distribution

India has the highest percentage of vegetarians 80% of the population or more than 40 million people. The world is definitely by vegetarian cities. law (prohibiting the consumption and presence of sales / meat found in their lands and in their surroundings slaughterhouses), most of them in India. They are holy cities Hinduism or Jainism: Pushkar, Haridwar, Rishikesh, Ayodhya, Palitana For example. Bodhgaya, holy city Buddhism At the request of Buddhist monks - and actor Richard Gere - A point of view can be a strict vegetarian area Legal.

In India, vegetarianism is common and has developed original business methods; India A country where more than a billion people live, where the percentage of vegetarian population is the most important. Many restaurants in India stand out - as well as markets, "non-vegetarian", "vegetarian" or "pure vegetarian" (expressing the lactose-vegetarian diet). According to Hindu-CNN-IBN 2006 31% of the Indians are lacto-vegetarians, and 9% are lacto-ovo-vegetarians: 40% of Indians are vegetarians in the western sense (no meat) and about 500 million people (ie, meatless). up population European union); However, a study of 2018 raises this figure to 20% as the proportion of households consuming meat increases. Among all communities, vegetarianism is the most popular diet. Hindus with almost 50% practitioner (between Jains Muslims (3% vegetarians), Christians (8% of vegetarians) and residents of coastal areas are 100% obligatory and less frequently required among fish consumers, respectively. Indian women are more likely to be vegetarians than men. Similarly, some Tamil Nadu's Although vegetarian fame, people in southern India are more likely than northern citizens largely western cliché. These same studies show that even meat-eating Indians are very rarely (less than 30% of regular consumers) because of the cost of these products. India created a visible label system for solid vegetarian products: a green dot in a green square. A "red dot inside a red square" sign indicates that the dish is definitely not a vegetarian. Medications are marked with a similar label: Omega-3 pill It is marked with "red dot on red square" because it uses non-vegetarian materials made of fish oils.

Nutrition balance

Vegetarianism is a diet that does not risk more than diet. eater diet If sufficiently diversified.

For vegans this diversity should mainly concern protein sources, rich in legumes lysine More than herbs. beans dry contact lenses Containing too much protein (21-24%) and soybean for example, beef has 17% to 35-37% protein: in fact, many plants containing protein bring more than meat.

Vegetarians and diets that consume a small amount of milk or egg products must supplement their purchase. Vitamin B 12 or through fortified foods B12 or with a dietary supplement. Depending on sunlight Vitamin D Supplement It may also be necessary. As with other diets nutritional deficiencies. In some foods the diet may occur if not sufficiently changed.

As with all diets, the contribution of vegetarian nutrition should mainly consist of proteins, carbohydrates and fats, as well as some substances such as small amounts of vitamins and minerals. Fiber they are not assimilated during digestion but participate in the smooth progress.

PROTEINS, CARBOHYDRATES, LIPIDS AND FIBERS

Proteins amino acids are small molecule polymers. There are twenty different amino acids that are said to be necessary in eight adult people (nine in babies). These required amino acids It cannot be synthesized from other molecules by the body and should be provided by the diet. Almost all proteins, whether animal or plant, contain twenty amino acids, in particular eight essential amino acids, but grains (wheat, rice, corn ...) tend to be low. lysine and isoleucine and legumes (beans, lentils, peas, chickpeas ...) are poor methioninem and tryptophan. However, there is a general: soy bean is a legume, but it is rich in methionine and is known for its high lignin corn varieties (such as opaque-2 diversity). .

Therefore, it is often recommended to combine cereals and legumes at a single meal; for example, to eat bread or pasta while eating lentils or peas. Traditional cultures did not expect nutritionists to discover and use the virtues of this mixture. Corn and beans in South America, rice and lentils in India, rice and soybeans in Southeast Asia, couscous and chickpeas in the Maghreb ... italian recipes in the country.

Various plant foods contain all important amino acids in good proportions, eg soybean, Kinoe, cannabis seeds and amaranths. Nutritional yeast (Saccharomyces cerevisiae especially rich in lysine; It can be eaten as a flake, but it also enters into the composition of many vegetable and salt spills (casserole...). Some nutritionists recommend that essential amino acids are present in sufficient amounts at each meal, otherwise protein synthesis is prevented; others feel it enough combination of essential amino acids performed in one day. American Dietetic Association "Only sources of vegetable protein can provide an adequate amount of amino acids if they are consumed in various ways and their energy needs are met."

Plants such as cereals, roots, fruits and vegetables are very rich. carbohydrates. Like any diet, it is necessary to minimize intake simple candies and in favor of intake slow candies. Indeed, simple sugars included sucrose called sugar commonly consumed sugar is likely to lead to the development of diseases such as weight gain and diabetes. However, most fruits are rich in simple sugars, but also bring in many vitamins and fibers. As a result, confections, jams, animal material may not contain, but nevertheless, due to simple sugar richness, they must be consumed in small amounts.

Contribution lipids It is not problematic as part of a vegetarian or vegan diet. Indeed, the only possible deficiency can come from the absolute absence Unsaturated fatty acids It is not called by the body because it is called the basic. This is for example linoleic acid. However, most vegetable oils provide adequate intake of these essential fatty acids. Vegetable origin oils are healthier for the body than for animals, because they prevent cardiovascular diseases. And avoid the onset of atherosclerosis.

It is essential for good progression of intestinal digestion, dietary fiber It is abundantly found in almost all fruits, vegetables and cereals.

Mineral Nutrients

Calcium found in all plants, especially in leafy sections; for example, spinach. Broccoli and other species cabbage also high. Oleaginous fruits Almond (plain or puree) and dried fruits FIG also rich in calcium. Commercial soy milk and soy yoghurt are usually supplemented with calcium in the same proportion as cow's milk (approx. 1200mg / 1). Some mineral waters, tap water in some regions is also an important resource. Oil seed purées, such as whole almond or sesame porridge, contain large amounts of calcium. Cow milk is a rich source for lactose-vegetarians. Good legumes like lentils, beans or peas Iron such as oil seed porridge (almond, sesame...), molasses or full sugar. Although not hememic, plant-derived iron is well absorbed by the body thanks to vitamin C. However, vegetarians are not immune to iron deficiency. weaken the immune system and calcium .

Algae and iodized salt are noteworthy sources. iodine In the diet. Plants are a random source, their iodine richness depends on the soil they grow. magnesium vegetables and fruits such as bananas and almonds. Sources manganese. Includes rice (mostly completed), avocado or eggs. Selenium It is found in mushrooms, chicory and garlic. In the vegetable world, zinc mostly found in walnuts and almonds. Also found in dairy products. Many trace elements, minerals and chemical elements, including fluorine, copper, chromium or bromine, are found in mineral or mineral water.

Vitamin deficiency and intake

C vitamin It is found in lots of fruits and vegetables. Vitamin D It is found in plants too, but is made by the skin when exposed to sunlight. Reinforcement may be recommended for children with darker skin (less vitamin D) and / or less sunlight, especially children. Vitamin D (vegetable origin) is also supplemented in some commercial foods. Lacto-ovo-vegetarians will also find them in dairy products and, to a lesser extent, eggs. Excellent in vegetable oils and wheat bran Vitamin E. Green vegetables and dairy products Vitamin K large quantities.

Provitamin A Many tubers are found in roots and roots, and turn into vitamin A in the intestinal walls. Den Vitamin B12, B vitamins are easily found in the plant kingdom. Vegetables, cereals, legumes and nuts contain good amounts.

Vitamin B12 (or cobalamin has approved bioavailability only when it comes from animal products such as meat, seafood, milk or eggs. To avoid deficiency, vegans should consume sufficient amounts of supplements or supplements and other vegetarian dairy products. Eggs are a very small source. Even for ovo-lacto-vegetarians, there is a risk of deficiency. In a typical Western diet, dairy products are often the main vegetarian source of B-vitamin. 12, supplements and fortified products outside.

Causes Of Vitamin B12 Lack

Normally, in the human body, two groups of bacteria can synthesize in large quantities Vitamin B 12 In the small intestine (Pseudomonas and Klebsiella sp.) But this vitamin is not absorbed by the body.

Deficiency Vitamin B12 it may be the result of a vegetarian diet or vegan (without all animal products) without reinforcement. liver Abundant source of vitamin B12 it may take several years to indicate the true initial symptoms of megaloblastic anemia (or macrocytosis). According to a 2001 German study, 1 out of 3 vegetarians and 2 out of 2 organs are missing.

All foods in the animal kingdom contain a sufficient amount of B12 Some plants contain enough. Some products include cereal patties, soft drinks or some soy milk, pot,vegemite... Some products, such as some algae, are sometimes offered as a good source of B vitamins. 12 . However, these green algae contain only or predominantly an inactive form of vitamin B. 12 (Inactive Corrinoid) Spirulina in the form of tablets meet the needs of vegan diet doesn't look likE . However, studies have shown a significant proportion of other algae. Active Vitamin B12 bioavailable cobalamin). An indian working and a Japanese study,the actual presence of vitamin B indicates 12 in Chlorella tablets as in nori or wash (Porphyra umbilicalis purple and green. However, it has been shown that nori consumption does not resolve vitamin B deficiency. So far no study could confirm the bioavailability of vitamin B12 From chlorella .

In a study conducted by Helga Refsum on the average 48-year-old, 204 Indian men, including 1/4 lactose-vegetarian, B vitamin 12 lack can also be observed among vegetarians who regularly eat eggs and poultry. The study found that only 10% of the subjects examined had a normal B-vitamin level. 12 and more seriously, 52% of the subjects had a real deficit. The authors of this study have now directed their research to a possible genetic origin of these deficiencies observed in B vitamins12. .

Results of vitamin B12 lack

In the long term, vitamin B12 lack bad for the body. The most common results are hematological disorders (Biermer anemia generalized fatigue, digestive disorders or neurological disorders. Rare cases of degeneration of the spinal cord have been reported. By training this deficiency, vegetarian and vegan diets are also aggravating factors in tuberculosis and may be in the case of DCS.

During pregnancy and lactation, it is essential to check the amount of vitamin

B12 available only in the mother's diet, because only stocks are not sufficient to meet the needs of the fetus. A newborn develops many shortcomings within a few months (growth retardation, muscle loss, visual impairment, social retardation ...). Other serious symptoms were observed: kwashiorkor (if there is a lack of protein), deep deficiency anemia, hypotonia mental retardation, hypotonia with a tendency to sleep, otitis with double holes, pneumopathy. Older people also follow B population because vitamin B12 more difficult to digest with age.

Personal motivations

The decision to become vegetarian may be a combination of reasons:

Health

According to John Robbins' book, Food Revolution vegetarians and vegans Living an average of 6 to 10 years longer than the rest of the population. Christian Mortensen, male dean of humanity from 1994 for 1998 It was a vegetarian. Numerous statistics and research shows that vegetarian diet reduces the risk of developing cardiovascular pathology exact cancers, osteoporosis, asthma, arthritis, diabetes and obesity. "While external factors such as physical activity and smoking and alcohol can play a role, an meatless diet is a clear contributor to reducing the morbidity and mortality of many chronic degenerative diseases," the American Dietetic Association said. it considers that vegetarian nutrition is effective for the prevention and treatment of many conditions. Too much consumption of meat and offal is also associated with its appearance. gout (deposition uric acid). The advantage of vegetarian and vegan diets, however, is not always evident when scientists compare them to non-vegetarian diets of individuals in health status. Austrian study it finds that vegetarians may have worse health (more cancer, allergy and mental problems, but less urinary incontinence) than non-vegetarians.

By Diet Guides for Americans, 2010 A report prepared by the Ministry of Agriculture and Health and Services. United States of America between America:

In their prospective adult studies, vegetarian-style eating habits with regard to non-vegetarian nutrition practices have been associated with better health outcomes: lower obesity, reduced risk cardiovascular disease, and death." total low. Some clinical studies have shown that vegetarian eating habits have decreased. Blood pressure. On average, vegetarians consume less amount. calorie from fat (especially saturated fat), less total calories, more fiber , potassium and C vitamin as non-vegetarian. Vegetarians generally have a lower body mass index. These characteristics and other lifestyle factors associated with a vegetarian diet may contribute to positive health outcomes detected in vegetarians.

Scientific activities in vegetarianism increased concerns about nutritional adequacy health and prevention disease. American Dietetic Association and Dietitians Canada They stated that a well-planned vegetarian diet at every stage of life is "healthy, suitable for nutrition and health benefits in the prevention and treatment of certain diseases". Large-scale studies have shown deaths caused by deaths. Ischemic heart disease vegetarians were 30% lower in males and 20% lower in vegetarian females than non-vegetarians. Vegetarian diets at low levels saturated fat, cholesterol and animal protein and higher levels carbohydrates, fiber, magnesium, potassium, folate and antioxidants as vitamin C and TO, and phytochemicals.

Some researchers like Dean Ornish treatment of heart disease in some patients with a strict vegetarian diet and stress. Nutritional concerns also encourage regimens that prefer fruits, vegetables and cereals, and minimize but not ban the absorption of meat and fats. Vegetarianism can lead to shortcomings Vitamin B12 and D or iron. However, the theory that large amounts of iron in animal foods can easily be absorbed is also controversial. In the case of proteins, they are found not only in meat but also in dairy products, eggs, bread, spirulina, cereals and So-called cereals as Kinoe oily fruits (almonds, walnuts, hazelnuts, pumpkin seeds, sesame seeds v) and legumes (beans, lentil, pea, chickpea, Soya beans).

Prevention of Cancer and Cardiovascular diseases

A research published in 2016 defines meat and milk protein consumption as a risk factor for mortality, but this relationship is only observed for patients with another risk factor (excess weight or obesity, high alcohol, smoking, sedentary lifestyle). Meat consumption will be an aggravating factor in the case of metabolic disorder.

Epidemiological studies Conducted by Prospective Research on the European Cancer and Nutrition (EPIC) network United Nations Human Development Report (2007-2008) and Harvard University In 2012, by An Pan and Frank Hu, meat eating (especially red meats and cold meats) increased the risk of cancer (four times more involved in the risk of death from cancer - the proteins consumed show that the plant was lost - Origin), Colon cancer (35% additional risk -Argentina and Most big red meat Uruguay , in the world Colon cancer) and gastric cancer, As well as cardiovascular diseases. Other studies classify flesh as one of the possible factors that prefer colorectal cancer. except for moderate consumption (50 g per day)

However, some meta-studies do not consider enough statistical data to conclude. Processed meat consumption (eg deli meats) and some cancers (colorectal, esophagus and stomach looks better established. Several studies have linked the carcinogenic effect of processed meats to the addition of preservatives. Nitrite fresh meat missing. Nitrites are the precursors of the carcinogenic family of compounds: nitrosamines. Exposure to nitrosamines as well as consumption of processed meat and fish, including smoked products - increases your risk gastric cancer. Consumption of acid salted water protected vegetables (such as pickled pickles) increases the risk of stomach cancer and esophagus they also contain large amounts of nitrosamine precursors.

There is also a link between red meat consumption or pancreas cancer can be accused without saturated fats; For authors, the effect of cooking on excessive risk should be investigated. The way meat is cooked as plant food plays an important role in carcinogenic potentials. Two compounds acrylamide and Method Criteria roast (roast) with high temperature cooking - cooking in contact with flames, especially for french fries) - especially for meat.

On October 26, 2015, the International Agency for Research on Cancer (a subsidiary of the WHO) exact carcinogen (group 1) and red meat as a possible carcinogen (group 2A) based on limited indications that cannot exclude the effect of other factors or a statistical illusion. .

Prevention of Alzheimer's disease

Given similarities symptoms (dementia and the causes of these serious pathologies Creutzfeldt-Jakob disease (human equivalent cattle spongy encephalopathy) and Alzheimer's disease (which one is two neurodegenerative diseases characterized by accumulation protein aggregate - in spite of different species - Forming degeneration At the brain level, some clinical studies tend to show consumption consumption. Meat (fish included) Large quantities Alzheimer's disease encourages development.

In particular, the role of methionine, which has been transformed into homocysteine by intermediate metabolism, is invoked in some studies. Hyperhomocysteinemia is a factor that increases the cardiovascular risk and appears to play a role in the onset of Alzheimer's disease. However, it is necessary to remember methionine one amino acid It is absolutely essential for life that does not cause any public health problems when consumed in the usual quantities. According to some theories, the increase in the number of cases Alzheimer's disease It may correspond to the increase in meat consumption in the world: Thus, a research American Nutrition Association On Populations, Latin America , from China and India concludes that meat consumption was high among the outgoing " diagnosis one dementia. In doing so, it implements vegetarianism. Indian The population (over the generations) has the proportion of individuals affected by Alzheimer's disease, the lowest rate recorded worldwide.

Prevention of cataracts

A 2011 study evaluated the relationship between diet and diet. Cataract risk in United Kingdom. For 15 years, 27,670 people were followed: the highest risk of developing cataracts was found in heavy consumers of animal meat. This risk is slightly reduced in the group consuming moderate amounts. For vegetarians and more vegans, risk reduction for cataract 40% bigger; This is to be linked Campbell Report defends studies showing which one is including in the diet found in colored vegetables carotenoids protects against macular degeneration which may cause eye disease blindness and containing a diet lutein, one antioxidant found in spinach provides protection against cataract.

Animal Welfare

Breeding and cutting conditions deteriorated

If Envas hayvan of domestic animals (aggressive animals as a result of treatment);

"Animal madness" means intense and long-term weakness, (chickens "in-between" pecking between the cages ablation (gives pain) beaks, pigs if not imprisoned stalls but in eden large en cages, Self-Mutilate , etc.);

And kinship the official definition of a non-relative individual, which leads to the physical or mental insufficiency (or fragility) of the farmer or "race" animals: parent there is no common ancestor in five generations [:] Have less and less animals he is not related today: economy. At the same tme did not block selection genetic poverty".

Animal rights

An application that can be motivated by vegetarianism law - A set of rules governing human behavior in society is defined as in social relations -. " in accordance with the law rights of animals.

Vegetarianism (or the ban on killing / eating an animal), as a norm to be applied by law antiquity with India, Emperor's Edicts Ashoka (v. 304 B.C). J. - C. - 232 B.C), in Gujarat the laws of the king Jain Gambling la (1143-1172), and Japan laws removed (676) AD.-C. By the Emperor temm of for example, also European under Pre-Socrates especially, Pythagoras and Empedocles:

"Cicero He critically compares the two philosophers [Pythagoras and Empedocles] in his eyes when he declares that they all live the same way. right the same sanctions were required murder and those who kill animals : men [...] create a community with animals, not just with the gods - skeptical Sextus Empiricus "Like a soul, a soul that permeates the whole cosmos Élisabeth de Fontenay, The Silence of Animals, Philosophy of Animation Test, Voltaire it also resembled against any shape Anthropocentrism and who justified respectful vegetation.

Today, the American philosopher Tom Regan, a professor North Carolina state University (and the head of American Value Inquiry Association In 1993 he is famous for advocating vegetarianism and animal law; firstly, taking into account the mental lives of animals, it takes support and participates in the development of the theory of law, which is considered by the degree of complexity:

The result of T. Regan is that some animals have a mentally complex life enough to accurately experience their well-being. In other words, they have a complex mental life that is so important to them.

In doing so, the results of this perspective lead to thinking of the animal. as such as Rights Handle:

Lar Beings that are the subjects of a life have a natural value. Only the language of rights can express the need not to harm themselves without compelling reasons. The subject of a life in which a person can demonstrate a mental complex so that he can deal with his well-being. Followed by these animals Which life of the subject, and they Which rights holders, even if they do not know this.

The obligations imposed by such a conception of law go beyond the practice of vegetarianism:

"Tom Regan as unfair practices or institutions, hunting , fishing , meat supply , circuses, zoos, intensive agriculture. At the same condemnation of experiments conducted on animals in also includes aspects of medical or biological. The only (in a carefully defined self-defense situation (without paying attention), he agrees with the principle of harm. To justify the protection of the owner of these rights, even before it is said to be the subject of a life, to give rights and to say what makes life precious. it is sufficient. to live. Public authorities should protect these rights independently of the neutral, good and evil conception."

This perspective is shared (but expanded to include all cognitive emotions and not only animals with complex cognitive abilities). Law professor at New Jersey State University- Gary Francione writes,:

The animal rights movement argues that all living beings have a right, whether human or not: the fundamental right of not being considered as the property of others . Our acceptance of this fundamental right means that we must remove it - not just regulation - they are animal exploitation practices. Suppose the animals are the property in humans, because each of us can take a main step towards the abolition, think that vegan lifestyles and educate the public about it the way of life . "

Therefore, this relationship with the law is related to human or non-human beings for the benefit of all one the understanding of justice; Therefore, Vegetarianism at the entrance to a lifestyle Dudley Giehl, Isaac Bashevis Singer writes:

"As long as mankind continues to pour blood into the animals, there will be no peace in the world. Creation of the distance between Hitler gas chambers and Stalin concentration camps are only a step away, because all these actions were carried out in the name of social justice , and the man to destroy the weaker beings than him. one knife or pistol unless it holds no justice will be . "

Likewise, Charles Patterson , Theodor W. Adorno , summarizing the idea of Eternal Treblinka writes:
"Auschwitz begins where everyone looks and thinks of a slaughterhouse: these are only animals. "
Therefore, refusing to see animals as lar machines eyen, but as emotional beings who do not want to be subjected to any pressure and want to live:

It is cruel and a barbarity to kill, destroy and slaughter the harmless animals , because if they say it in a bad, wrong and absurd way, they are also vulnerable to evil and suffering. The new Cartesians are soulless and pure machines without any emotions. If you don't see it, you clearly tend to suppress within the absurd opinion, since the heart of the pernicious and the disgusting doctrine of the hearts of all men among the emotions that poor animals can have for courtesy , courtesy and humanity. We must surely believe that they are as sensitive as they are sensitive to good and evil, that we have the pleasure and the pain, that we are our servants, and that life and work are our faithful companions and that they are treated gently. Blessed are the Gentiles with kindness and goodness you treat them and their miseries and pains of sympathy, but who is cursed by treating them cruelly nations persecuted them love their pouring blood who is willing and dinner. their flesh. Jean Meslier, Folie men, attribute the brutal and barbarian victims of innocent animals to the institution and believe that such victims are their tastes.

Or:
"Humanity against lower animals is one of the most noble virtues of man and is the final stage of the development of moral sentiments." However, when we are concerned about the sum of our living beings, our morality has reached the highest level. The animals we built like us are suffering from our savages very often. The one who did not have the motives, the suffering of the animals, the barbaric action, would say something of the inhumanity, because it would torture a flesh, and our sister savages a body that shares the same mechanism of life with us. Same ability for pain. "

Ethic vegetarians ya think that the majority of the world's population is fed only with tradition, comfort, habit or pleasure. These reasons do not seem enough to cause them suffering from meat production in agreement with Rabindranath Tagore . (Nobel Prize for Literature in Asia in 1913 , said:

Uz We eat animal flesh because we don't think about the persecution of this action. "

This type of vegetarianism is often associated with the animal liberation movement , although not all ethical vegetarians subscribe to the concept of animal rights. However, since this Code of Ethics, it may have another philosophical source; So, the philosopher and priest of Apollon most Delphi, Plutarch and Latin poet Ovid (Referring to Pythagoras, he treats vegetarianism ethically:

For a small meat, the life, the sun, the light from them and we take the flow of a life in the forefront of nature: we think that the screams they throw through fear are not expressed, they mean nothing. For each of these poor moaning animals just There are prayers, prayers and justifications. We look indifferent to a loss of soul? I want Empedocles not to be what they believe, father, mother, son or friend ; it is always an entity that feels, sees, hears, hears, hears, he has the intelligence and intelligence to obtain the appropriate ones for each animal and avoid damaging him / her. "

Plutarch , if meat is allowed to eat .

One day human blood, a coil of one prepares to cast "How awful, tastes lamb in cold blood, and his plaintive bleatings is an insensitive ears; he who can kill mercilessly young goat and hear wailing as her child; you can eat Who birds! Fed in the hands of this long Is there a way to end criminal offenses, murder? Isn't it clear? Let oxen plow and die only from old age; LED sheep brought us icy breath against Boreas and The goats put their full breasts in the hands pressing them. No more features and no lake, no traitor; Do not scratch the bird on the glue, do not put the scared deer into your canvases, do not hide the point of the hook under a deceptive oath.

Ovid , Metamorphoses , book XV .
Antispécisme is a philosophical and political movement that believes that all emotional beings (that can feel pain, pleasure and other emotions and emotions) are morally equal; and as a result, the interest of a non-human animal in a happy and satisfying life is as important as his or her equal interests. Therefore, according to this movement, speciesism is an arbitrary discrimination based on species, as well as racism based on gender racism. and discrimination based on sexism based on arbitrary discrimination. In this regard, the famous philosopher utilitarist Peter Singer, philosopher from quotations doing the Black Code, which refers Jeremy Bentham between Louis XIV governing slavery

"The French , the darker the skin, without a possible plea to the whims of one who tortured him that there was no reason for the abandonment of a man already discovered. One day, the number of claws , villus skin or termination are sufficient reasons for leaving the body susceptible to the same fate of the sacrum bone . a dog or an adult horse , beyond all possible comparison , a day of innovation , a week's or a month is a more rational beings and are more suitable for speech . But what would have followed if they were otherwise? The real question is," Can they make a reason or not?" However: "May I suffer?

Jeremy Bentham, Introduction to Moral and Legislation Principles (17d. 1780). Peter Singer's expression "A chimpanzee or eg pig , new born one A baby is much closer to the autonomous and models to be rational based "and claiming that asserts the argument reveals:" extensive brain damage, which attracts not appropriate to accept the life of a child abandoned in a similar mental level one dog or a pig unacceptable to kill. The interest of addressing evenly and equal treatment "this last claim, which is linked to a parallel debate has provoked a distinction between, especially in Christian circles caused several polemics and criticism.

With the criticism of post-trade "mode plus a large, a certain development social sciences born on the peninsula, and Claude Levi-Strauss , for example, is not the most famous:

"Now Rousseau's idea of the ability to detect the use of human virtues in a non-owner humanism flaws open to hit , what we think, unfortunately in ourselves that we can observe ! and lethal effects for ourselves ... Because of the nature itself , a first destruction that must inevitably follow another mutilation to undergo causing the myth of the exclusive dignity is not it? We started by cutting off the people of nature. In her ruling a rule establishing, most undeniable character, so everything before that creature was believed to erase . You are blind to this city that you will not abuse. Jamais better knowledge father des quatre derniers century de son of the shirt histoire ballet her deception queen s'arrogeant comprendre Le droit de séparer radicalement Carmack's animalité, He refused to hear another clerk in accordant to ce qu we heard, cursed circle and the other frontier, the civil servant was recaptured, served as the guardian of other homosexuals, and revitalized at the expense of minorities, and the limiting privileges of a degenerated humanism that wasted the abomination of Aussitôt.

Other motivations, the more precise, the definition of ethics, the principle is the cause of the majority of vegetarianism for humanity that imposes non-existent violence , such as the Hindu (original "non-violence", or majority ahimsa , basic Manuu laws by Hindu life policy in society is synonymous with vegetarianism/veganism/veganism) or a request to revalue death and suffering until unimportant :

"All this talk of dignity, compassion, culture or morality, of those who kill innocent creatures, the foxes that are consumed by their mouths , and even of the bullfights. And it seems ridiculous when it comes out of the mouth of those who encourage the existence of slaughterhouses . All these explanations are hypocrites, according to which nature is ruthless and therefore we have the right to be ruthless. Nothing can prove a man is more important than a butterfly or a cow . . I'm thinking of being the vegetarian of my life. I do not claim to have saved many animals from the slaughterhouse, but my refusal to eat meat protests the persecution ... Personally, I do not believe that as long as animals are treated as they are today, there is no peace in this world . "

Environmental interes

Battery farming least one surface, or livestock outdoor pets (rare) (eg, food require in larger quantities, but single culture) amount grown on land (meat consumption is increasing worldwide, requiring the forests): 38% of the Amazon forest destroyed beef cattle 247 and at least 100 species are disappearing every day because of the forest 247 "extinction of species main reason mostly high density, for example, attributed the loss in endemic areas Brazilian jungle or in the forests of Madagascar , which reduced 90% of its original size over the last forty years.

Food for breeding and fattening cattle use 78% of global agricultural land

A hectare of growing fruit and vegetables can feed up to thirty people with a soil, but if the same hectare is used to produce eggs or white meat, it can feed only five people, and if one person only produces red meat, it is less than. One kilogram of animal protein 250 makes 7 to 10 kg of herbal protein.

Fight against overfishing

Fishing and Troll is also harmful to marine ecosystems and to biodiversity that has taken place over tens of thousands of years. In doing so, 90% of large fish (Tuna, swordfish, Atlantic swordfish, codfish, tuna fish, skates and flounder is over hunting and is therefore in danger .

In addition, the troll condemned the deaths of other marine mammals and birds , and the turtles and fish were crushed, but unnecessary, as was the case with the original animal species in which they were caught and broken. Faut-il manger des animaux in his book , Jonathan Safran Foer notes:

In the case of shrimp, other sea animals 13 kg for 500 grams . In other non-target species, killed in tons of fish, which were killed and discarded, regularly killed, especially dolphins, which are usually killed on tuna, dolphins thus killed ground in cranes with tuna.

Natural Resources Economics

The World Watch Institute considers that the current amount and the future is probably not sustainable in terms of production of meat and animal products in the future sustainable development in order to the environment . John Mayer, nutritionist between Harvard University , the US meat consumption in the case of a 10% drop, US agriculture about 60 million people in the world can feed cereals and vegetables estimates .

Water is becoming an increasingly scarce resource in many parts of the world. Excessive consumption by humans damages rivers and ecosystems and causes salinity and desertification. A vegetarian diet consumes less water than a meat-based diet.

Fight against global warming

Animal protein requires eight times more fossil fuel expenditure than comparable amounts of plant protein . This fossil fuel consumption one produces greenhouse gas, carbon dioxide. Animal production is also one Although compost produces fertilizer base, it releases methane . Within the United States (the world's largest greenhouse gas transmitter) livestock produces approximately 20% of total methane emissions. A ton of methane, 23 tons of carbon dioxide has a global warming potential.

The vegetarian diet will also be a way of fighting against global warming: the rate for a pound of meat production is 100 times greater than producing the same amount of grain . Cows such as cows produce 100 grams of methane daily , 25 times that of CO one has the potential to warm up.

It is estimated that global livestock production produces more greenhouse gases than all transport (land, air, sea) in the world," a report published by FAO (UN agricultural agency). Considering the whole production chain of meat, it represents 18% of the emissions of these human-produced gases.

One of the main causes of global warming . According to Frank Mitloehner, this study may be prejudiced that it will compare a taşımacılık global "estimate of livestock-related emissions with a non-global estimate of transport-related emissions. However, he admits that this figure can be globally definitive

In May 2009, Ghent was "the first vegetarian in the world at least once a week" when local authorities decided to establish a "week-free day". Officials, political figures and various officials would accept vegetarian food one day a week by accepting this UN report. Public posters encouraged people to take part in şehir vegetarian days m and printed city maps showing vegetarian restaurants. From September 2009, the city will be one of the schools and ggiedag ("vegetarian day") weekly .

Solidarity of Peoples

One of the arguments put forward by some vegetarians is the moral solidarity with the peoples of the Third World and the exploited men. During the direct, during the famine (more than a million deaths), as in 1985, the local population (while it is used for consumption, in fact, the cereals that go to the feeding of the western cattle continue to export cereals for the British cattle fattening in Ethiopia, which are generally grown in third world countries):

The world can feed 1.5 billion disinfected people every year with one billion tonnes of grain feeding animals for the massacre . If all North Americans avoid meat-eating once a week, they indirectly feed 25 million poor people every day for a year! It will also help to tackle climate change effectively. Therefore , according to Rajendra Kumar Pachauri , the Nobel Peace Prize winner [...] is a global vegetarian-oriented global trend, which is essential to combat the worst in the world, the shortage of energy and the impact of climate change. Including in our concerns, the fate of other species is in no way compatible with the determination to do the best we can to solve human problems. The protection of animals and the weakest man is the same right to help those who may be harmed . "

According to Fabrice Nicolino , regular meat supply is only possible for a minority person with sufficient income to buy: but such a diet is impossible to spread to the world, and the increase in the population of people suffering from starvation is a scandal. because, at the same time, the fattening of a maximum animal subject when grown for meats:

But No people have ever been affected by famine. There are more than a billion people today. At the same time, meat consumption also explodes. [...] When we know that making a kilogram of vegetable protein takes 7 to 10 kilos, there is the question of where to feed herds from animal proteins . We have to choose between feeding people or animals.

According to the Ministry of India 's agriculture , one hectare of arable land can produce 20 tons of potatoes against only 50, kgof meat. In India, vegetarian nutrition is considered to be one of the solutions to malnutrition, but factory agriculture and large landowners' lobbies are advancing in the opposite direction.

Desmond Morris, Plutarch follows the tracks and Montaigne, the obligation of respect for animals , the citizens of democratic countries, to operate as slaves or that they will make most of the behaviors they allow themselves to be unbearable against other men they are hungry for; Which Milan reflects the passage of Kundera in Unbearable Lightness of Existence.

"There is no right to be nice with a boyfriend. (Iz) We cannot determine precisely what our relations, feelings, charity or hatred are, and to what extent. They are pre-conditioned by the balance of power between individuals: the true goodness of man can be shown only by those whose purity and freedom are not represented by any force. The true moral test of humankind (the level which is deep enough to escape from our most radical view), its relationship with what is at its mercy: the animals . that the basic bankruptcy of man occurred, so that the others are also caused by it."

Taste of meat

Some people do not like the taste of meat and cause the consumer. . Conversely, some foods for vegetarians try to increase the taste or texture of the meat (Tempeh, Seitan , tofu ready, textured soybean) .

(Due to a large portion of vegetarians worldwide, a vegetarian family in the world Vegetarians Hindu vegetarianism do not like the taste of usually meat) (meat first feeding can be followed by the vomiting) and animal baked smell of meat (mammals, birds, fish, etc.) Is very unpleasant for born vegetarian: this is because the palate and the senses firstly develop their abilities and preferences in childhood, and in doing so they take the vegetarian children.

More pleasure in consuming unloved vegetables by some children born in a meat-eating family . Mahatma Gandhi , during his youth, was convicted with a comrade and nationalist conviction. Meat he was persuaded to eat the goat (the British who ruled the Indians according to his friends for eating the flesh): it did not give him any pleasure, and he showed his nightmares where he was, and he saw the reincarnated goat killed by a butcher.

Animalists for vegetarians belonging to childbirth" because the idea of being next to someone to cook meat is discouraging" or antispecists , buildings in India, Mumbai in In particular, we offer apartments in private homes. areas where only vegetarians are allowed to live.

Some people think that meat is not appetizing, especially raw, and opts to avoid eating animal meat only for aesthetic or emotional reasons. Others will find the simple reality of being a vegetarian. In addition, some vegetarians believe a vegetarian-fed vegetation has a better body odor.

Religions

Religions of Indian origin.

Many religions, including Buddhism, Hinduism (especially in yoga the philosophy) Jainism and Sikhism Teach that all life must have value and must not be deliberately destroyed for unnecessary human gratification.

Hinduism

The ahimsa is the philosophical notion of Indian religions (of Hinduism, the Buddhism and Jainism) which introduces vegetarianism as a standard in the diet. Ahimsa is a value that recommends non-violence and respect for all life, be it human, animal or vegetable (since it is between Bishnoi). Ahimsa This very often results in non-violence or non-harm to all living beings or in respect for life in all its forms. The Sanskrit root is him ("hurt") with the privative "a". Ahimsa is based on a Vedic injunction: mahimsyat sarva-bhutani- that no living being is damaged. In the context of Hinduism, the term Ahimsa appears for the first time in the Upanishad and Raja Yoga. This is the first of five. yama or eternal votes, the essential restrictions of yoga (ahimsa does not lead to any specifically yogic state, but it is considered the first moral step essential for any "honest man). To this respect, Bhishma says in the Mahabharata:

"Is it necessary to say that these innocent and healthy creatures are made for the sake of life, when they want to be killed by miserable sinners who live in butchery? For this reason, O monarch, O Yudhishthir, you must know that the rejection of the flesh is the greatest refuge of religion, heaven, and happiness. Refraining from doing harm is the fundamental principle. Here again, it is the greatest penance. It is also the greatest truth among all the trials of affection. Meat can not be removed from grass, wood or stone. Unless a living being is killed, it can not be done. Then you miss meat. This man, who abstains from eating, is never afraid of him, O king. By no creature. All creatures require protection. He never causes anxiety in others, and he himself should never be. If no one eats meat, there is no one left to kill sentient beings. The man who kills living beings kills them for the sake of the one who eats meat. If the meat is considered inedible, there is no slaughter of living beings. Whoever eats meat has every interest in the killing of living beings in the world. Since then, oh, you are of great splendor, life is shortened for people who kill living beings or are the cause of their death. It is clear that the person who wants his property must completely abandon the consumption of meat. The buyer of the meat realizes the violence for its wealth: the one who eats the meat thus profits to savor its flavor, the murderer realizes that it attaches and kills the animal. So, there are three ways to kill. Whoever brings or brings the meat to himself, the one who cuts the limbs of an animal and the one who buys it, sells it, or the cooks of the meat and the one who eats it, all these things must be considered as meat eaters.

Belief in reincarnation is fundamental in the philosophical developments of Jainism, Buddhism and Hinduism, and in this belief system, souls (atman, animates "breath", principle of life, consciousness) can be embodied in the form of plants, animals or human beings. CNN He reports that 85% of the Indian population has a vegetarian diet. (no meat, fish or eggs, eggs are considered non-vegetarian foods in India). The diet, which relies mainly on dairy and organic foods, is practiced in Orthodox communities in southern India, in some northern states. Gujarat or from south to Karnataka where the influence of Jains It is significant. Some avoid onion and garlic considered to have Rajas properties, that is to say, "passionate". the svadharma (thestaff Dharma) Brahmins includes vegetarianism, Brahman is called to lead an absolutely pure life. Hinduism promotes vegetarianism. The consumption of meat, fish (and fertilized eggs) is not encouraged, it is only tolerated, it is tolerated in the framework assigned to it by Hinduism since the Vedas: inferior, non respectful with the. Some Brahmans are also vegans and do not consume any animal products (milk, etc.). Since the century Before Jesus Christ, the Upanishad Emphasize that animals and humans are brothers because they host all Atman and so are the sanctuaries of Brahman. In this religious conception, all living beings considered as sanctuaries of Atman, no temple of Atman is dedicated to him, unlike other deities such as Vishnu o Shiva . In most Hindu holy cities, it is forbidden to use non-vegetarian foods and alcohol, and it is forbidden by law to sacrifice the cows in almost all states of India. The leather However, a dead cow of natural origin is accepted.

Jainism

All food standards cited for Hindus apply to Jains. In addition to prohibiting the consumption of eggs, fish or meat, they must take into account the discomfort caused to plants and animals. Suksma Jiva (Sanskrit: subtle life forms who will then be called microorganisms) in your food options. According to the doctrine of the sect or branch of Jainism to which they belong, some Jainas avoid consuming most of the vegetable roots, such as potatoes, onions, etc. (some branches of Hinduism also eliminate onions, etc.) tamasic).

Buddhism

Schools of Buddhism (mahāyāna to in particular, to ask its followers to be at least vegetarian, the other Buddhist schools do not impose vegetarianism, but advise it; it is nevertheless at the Buddha to whom we owe the strengthening of this practice in India, through Emperor Ashoka. According to Vinaya (Theravada monastic code), monks are required to eat all the food they are given, including meat (but they do not eat them either: Buddhist monks should encourage vegetarianism- Nonviolence animals), except when the animal has been slaughtered by them or is on the list of prohibited animals (human, elephant, horse, dog, snake, Lion, Tiger, panther, bear) and hyena) Recently, Tibetans They profoundly change their eating habits and become more and more vegetarians. They follow the advice of the 14th Dalai lama and the 17th Karmapa in 2007 and 2008, he gave instructions on the benefits of not eating meat so as not to make animals suffer. It is noted that the Dalai Lama is not strictly vegetarian, since he contracted hepatitis B and damaged his liver, he had to follow the recommendations of the doctors who recommended him to eat meat. However, it limits its consumption and is considered semi-vegetarian. In the Tibet Autonomous Region, and in Kham and Amdo, open vegetarian restaurants.

Chinese religions

In Chinese societies, normal, old"Food" means a diet associated with Taoist monks and sometimes practiced by people at Taoist festivals. The term used to describe these practitioners is translated as "vegetarians". This diet rejects meat, eggs and milk, but that includes oysters and their derivatives.

According to Orthodox Taoist Canon (0179):

"This is the third precept: do not kill one animal for the food; instead, we must be caring and beneficial to everyone, including insects and towards."

Abrahamic religions

There is a long debate about the original nutritional practice of humanity. the Judaism, the Christianity, the Rastafarianism and Islam. They have a common cultural background in the history of humanity: Genesis, unique in the Bible. Indeed, in Genesis, two texts, of different orientation, mention the consumption of meat in the Garden of Eden:

"Master the fish of the sea, the birds of the sky and all the animals that move on the earth. I gave you all the herbs that carry their seed in the earth and all the trees that contain in them their seed according to their type, so that they serve you food. " - Genesis I, 28-29

"Feed on everything that has life and movement: I abandoned all these things, like vegetables and field herbs. "- Genesis, IX, 3

Divergent excerpts, additional interpretations are made in the history of humanity: from relatively early, you have to start a new tournament in the world. Ten seventh and eighth century, as a result of the publication in 1663 of Hierozoicon sive of bipartitum opus animibalus Sacrae Scripturae by Samuel Bochart, affirming the idea that Adam and Eve were consumed from the oldest ramp. Agustín Calmet wrote an audio commentary. Literary Literature of the Sciences of Man and the New Testament (1724) to refute the idea proposed by Bachart: according to him, "The fertility of the earth, the beauty of plants, the strength of time of men and the little kingdom, as well as the scarcity of animals in the Garden of Eden, led humans to set aside the absorption of meat. Doctors, naturalists, philosophers and historians have been in charge of proposing new questions.

Moreover, if you take into account the original in Hebrew Bible Without anthropocentric interpretations (according to some theologians, God would have made man only for men) Genesis nowhere indicates that animals need to be guided or directed to fulfill their destiny, which in fact praises God in their own way (Psalms, CXLVIII: 10). In primitive Judaism, Adam and his successors, the vegetarian, dominate fish and birds on an order of concept and not of practice. The title of ruler of animals is only honorary.

"Catholic" or anthropocentric interpretations were influenced by:

The Fathers of the Church, who fought against the belief in metempsychosis (in relationship with Manicisme, Pythagoras, Empedocles, pharisaism) the Neoplatonism This induces a break between human beings and other creatures.

And metaphorical connections between demons and beasts. (the snake The original sin he identified himself rather late with the devil, that the Genesis I was not).

For the followers of the holy poet. Kabir (which are 9.6 million), Bible (which is also one of his sacred books, the Koran, the Vedas, the Puranas and the Bhagavad Gita), orders to be vegetarian.

In Islam, Here not ban on being vegetarian (The latter then eats perfectly halal), although this practice is still rare in the Muslim world; However, vegetarianism is gaining adherents in Arab and Muslim countries. because it's not halal to raise an animal like a machine, and animals also deserve compassion, for they are, as men, creatures of God. I love Christianity and Judaism Islam claims that God created animals. But unlike Christianity, Islam is very interested in animals : In Animals in Islam Al-Hafiz Basheer Ahmad Masri, who was the Magnet from Shah Jahan Mosque to Woking, United Kingdom, from 1964 to 1968, he writes:

In fact, according to Koran (21, 107), Muhammad He was sent as "help of all creation. Some objections to vegetarianism in Islam could come from the fact that a practice like Eid el-Kebir it is incompatible with vegetarianism; Masri responds: "At the beginning of Islam, the tradition of offering animals made sense. Meat was then an essential ingredient of human nutrition and the crumb was not lost. Today, killing [animals] has become a meaningless ritual and the deep meaning [of the act] has been forgotten. Furthermore, Soheib Bencheikh great Mufti of Marseilles, believes that the sacrifice of sheep on the occasion of Eid al-Kebir, "it is neither a pillar of Islam, nor an important obligation comparable to the pray quick Ramadan"; He adds that the Islamic law allows to replace this act by "a gift made in a country where the inhabitants do not eat their hunger, which is more in keeping with the spirit of sharing than this practice. Involved Moreover, when we know that agriculture produces most of its grain production to fatten animals, but that humanity suffers from hunger and malnutrition in the world.

In addition, there is a tradition of vegetarianism in Islam, linked in particular to sufism. Great sufi saints from the past, they were vegetarians, like Mirdad, who said: "Those who follow the spiritual path must never forget that if they consume meat, they will have to pay for that gesture of their own flesh. " The lessons of Muslim indian and holy poet Kabir of Inayat Khan and the from Sri Lanka Bawa Muhaiyaddeen encourage vegetarianism. Historian William Montgomery Watt says that the kindness of Muhammad For animals, it was remarkable given the social context of their education. He cites a case in which Muhammad sent sentinels to ensure that the dog with his newborn puppies was not disturbed by the movement of his army to Mecca in the year 630.

It is said that Muhammad said (according to Umar and Abdullah Ibn al-As): "No man who kills even a sparrow or something smaller, act with merit, and Wing I asked him about it [the day of judgment] and "He who pleases the creatures of God, pleases him." . Muhammad also said, "For the good work given to every creature with a wet [ie, living] heart, there is a reward." Muhammad opposed sports hunting and said: "Trying to kill a living being for sport is a curse."

Both in the Sunita and Shiite texts, we note the fact that Muhammad spoke nonchalantly with camels, the birds and other animal species. Shiite texts extend this gift to include imams. In one hadeeth, we say that camel I manage to complain that, despite the devoted service he rendered to his landlord, he was about to be killed. Mohammed called the owner and ordered the man to save the camel. It is reported in the Koran it Solomon He spoke to the ants and the birds Ismaili Imams and Shiites declare that they can communicate with everything that has a soul, a life, all creatures. As members of sufism the holy poet Kabir consider that Muhammad He was a vegetarian, but that mullahs did not follow his example (the Mullah's law is not for Kabir the law of the Wing) .

Christianity

For fans of the Orthodox Church where the Churches of the three councils. such as Coptic Orthodox Church there are many long periods during which the feeding of products of the animal kingdom is strictly forbidden (veganism) and even to dress or use any product of the animal kingdom (veganism). On the other hand, unlike Orthodox Christianity, for example Catholicism (Opposed to Catharisme) eliminates all food bans (whether Jewish (eg pork) or pagan (Egyptians) the wise men and many other idolaters avoided killing and eating sheep, Goats, oxen). Around 560, the first panties board Declared in his fourteenth canon: "If anyone shares the doctrine of Mani and Priscillian, observe the impure flesh that God has created for our food and do not dare to taste vegetables even cooked with meat, let it be anathema." Then some the orders Christians (the Trapistas, the Chartreux, the Benedictine, the Parents of the desert and all the monastic orders of Orthodox Christianity), esoteric Christianity as the Rosicrucian Fraternity Christian anarchism (represented for example by Leo Tolstoy), but also the currents of Christianity like those of Cathars and Seventh-day Adventists, promotes vegetarianism.

Remember that the Vegetarian Society, the first vegetarian (de facto vegan) worldwide, was founded in 1847 by evangelical The Christians in Britain (student, Gandhi United). When vegetarianism is based on a Christian perspective, Biblical references are often the same as those of the following Jews and Rastafarians (from the Jewish messianic era (vegan) is for Christians and Rastafarians Jesus In the ground).

Judaism

According to some Tora scientists as rabbis Bonnie Koppel, Rami Shapiro and Yitzhak HaLevi Herzog, former Chief Rabbi of Israel God's original purpose was for man to be vegetarian, for vegetarianism is the ultimate meaning of the teaching of biblical morality. For them, God he then allowed men to eat meat because of their weakness (the propensity to commit murder as part of their new nature), but the ideal or the final will of God for men would be to be vegetarian. The Bible also states that man can eat sacrificed animals, but according to the ritual rules of sacrifice (in Judaism and Islam), if not kill an animal is a murder.

For the Bible, God has allowed Consumption of the flesh (because there were no plants, according to the Polish rabbi Yitzhak Hebenstreit, in his book Kivrot Hata'avah) Following the Flood respect, with regard to Judaism (and Islam), always prohibitions and rules of food embodied by Kashrut which indicate a great complication in the consumption of meat (the number of which is limited), the Tanach (Old Testament) evokes, in addition to prudence, the certainty of the final destiny of creatures:

Moreover, after the flood, God stated the noachide laws (valid for all men) which forbids the consumption of a quarter of the meat obtained at the cost of a mutilation, a vivisection. Moses Maimonides in his book the roaming guide, remember also in this regard that it is the concern for the physical suffering and "morality" of the animal that reflects these sacred rules.

About Talmud (Avodah Zorah 18b) which says: "Great importance is attached to the humane treatment of animals, the basic and human virtue is declared", Rabbi Samson Rafael Hirsch in Horeb, he adds: "You are here faced with the teaching of God, which requires you not only not to inflict suffering on an animal, but to help it and, when you can, to reduce suffering when you see an animal that suffers, even if it's not your fault. For some people The Jews Given the reduction in the number of animals in the state of "things" or "production machinery" in the current state of the world, with all that that implies, vegetarianism/veganism he is seen as a mitzvah facto. So, the former chief rabbi of Ireland Rabbi David Shlomo Rosen - He's a vegetarian himself - he believes it's forbidden to eat meat today halakha :
"The cruelty of today's treatment of animals in the cattle trade makes meat consumption absolutely unacceptable, the halachic perspective as a product of illegitimate means. "Franz Kafka On the other hand, he gave a vegetarian interpretation of the Bible in these terms.

Moses He led the Jews across the desert to not get used to eating meat during those forty years. the mana, vegetarian diet.

"The essential points of the Jewish conception of life they are as follows: affirmation of the right to life for all creatures; the life of the individual has sense only in the service of embellishing and ennobling the existence of all living beings; Life is sacred, that is, the supreme value upon which all evaluations rest. "

Albert Einstein, In my eyes, the Jewish ideals.

Anyway, the reign of Messiah (Isaias, 11) announcement for some renowned rabbis, such as Rav Kook and Isaac Arama (and for Rastafarians and Black Hebrew) a return to vegetarianism /veganism. Around the world and practiced before Flood, vegetarianism even extends to creatures considered carnivorous (as in Original paradise, Genesis: I: 30), to give rise to the spectacle of a universal fraternity.

The opinions

The moralization of a food practice.

If criticism of high levels of meat consumption in Western societies is justified, the absolute prohibition of vegetarianism from consuming meat is, as any absolute, considered by some to be a moral vision and, as such, can be subject to the classic critics of morality. Imperatives (universalistic temptations, potential intolerance, etc.). According to the philosopher. Dominique Lestel vegetarians in the line of antispecies (and Hinduism, Jainism and Buddhism), they separate from "the animality" making the human being the only omnivorous Refuse the consumption of meat that causes suffering related to breeding or slaughter, while the man who eats meat would assume an "animal" nature. Although the term "animal" has been challenged by the philosopher Jacques Derrida in his book The animal I am , where there is the idea that man is not a "robot" who must follow a "program" because he can (It must be omnivorous, because its organism allows it: culturally, the meats consumed are different, there are slaughterhouses for dogs and the cats in China For example, the practice of cannibalism in Papua New Guinea. The rejection of the consumption of meat products by Jews and Muslims, the consumption of insects in food is almost non-existent in Europe but not in Asia, etc.), but it is a cultured animal ("deferred nature") who builds his human universe in relation to his own understanding of the world around him and still constitutes it - nature ("deferred culture") - because he wants it (philosopher Elisabeth de Fontenay in The silence of animals, considers that any definition of "own man" or "nature or human essence" is dangerous (and only of European origin), excluding those which do not conform to this definition minor humanity, bringing them closer to the often unenviable destiny of "the animal", a term too general to be valid from the philosophical point of view).

A food practice perceived as unnatural.

Vegetarianism is sometimes perceived as contrary to the nature of the human species.

The human species has evolved control the fire and tools to hunt and cut meat, reducing stress on teeth and claws. Since the development of stone tools, prehuman species have begun to consume meat. 2 million years ago. Since human beings have co-evolved with their tools, we can not rely on an analysis of our anatomy without taking into account this parameter. Since the beginning of Homo erectus, Adaptation to the consumption of meat with the help of tools and the fire is manifested: reduction of the size of the intestine, weakening of the teeth and increase of the size of the brain. Unlike the great apes left in the forest, savanna prehumans have had to adapt: fruits and seeds are rare in the savannah, but not the large herbivores relatively easy to hunt. Our ability to digest meat was acquired by natural selection during the period. The consumption of proteins (animal or vegetable) was very advantageous: rich in nutrients dense energy, sustained brain growth and maintained good athleticism despite increased height. Since 1.5 million years, meat consumption. It's regular with our ancestors. These anatomical and palaeontological observations confirm the omnivorous character of the human species and The importance of meat in the evolution of our species.

However, as "omnivorous" (able to "eat everything") is the human species, we must not forget that humans have chosen to abstain (for example, India, of the tempspréhistoriques as shown in Jainism and Hinduism), or to abstain from such or such meat for usual reasons (the cats and dogs you can eat like meat in China, not in Europe) or religious (no consumption of pigs   of   20 insects and Raptors , etc. , in the Jewish World or Muslim, as part of the biblical Koranic orders) The human being is never totally "omnivorous". in fact (except in the case of cannibalism). For vegetarianism, it's a cultural practice, and against nature. Vegetarianism is not an "anomaly" in human "nature", since it is a cultural choice (for example, abstaining from eating meat). dog a cat , etc) who practices .

Some thinkers still argue that the human being is obliged, by its very nature, to be a vegetarian, In particular, confident in the fact that teeth Among humans, medium-strength mandibles and small canines are not sharp, they are comparable to those of frugivorous primates (which, if they consume meat occasionally, are inherently frugivorous), without taking into account the fact that we evolved with tools and fire. They make our teeth less decisive; so Charles Darwin to declare:

"The classification of forms, organic functions and diets clearly showed that the normal food of human beings is vegetable in the same way as that of anthropoids and monkeys , this hour canines They are less developed than theirs and we do not intend to compete with wild or carnivorous animals. We have seen that the senses and intuitions, different emotions and faculties, such as love and memory attention and curiosity Limitation The reason, etc., of which the human being boasts, can be found in the nascent state or even fully developed in the lower animals. Animals, of which we have made our slaves, we do not like to consider them as our equals.

Charles Darwin, From the origin of species to natural selection.   .

Recent scientific research indicates that the emergence of agriculture 10,000 years ago may have fostered the genetic evolution of humans, allowing them to incorporate more vegetables into their diets. .

"The wise do not kill animals" said Porphyry; Only barbarians kill and eat them. - Voltaire, The dialogue of capon and chicken

Unlike herbivores and eating seeds, humans do not possess culture or one The belly specific use exclusive fodder and other foods rich in cellulose, his intestine it is ten to twelve times the length of its body, a typical size of omnivores such as pork and bear, four to five times in carnivores and twenty times in cattle .

Voltaire, in his writing Marseille and the lion He considered that animal meat was not the natural food of the human being since, with "his puny teeth" and his "weakness". stomach", this one" could not only, without the art of a cook, / Digest a chicken. So Georges Cuvier, Charles Giraud o Charles Darwin among others) considered frutarism as the most naturally adapted to the physiology of human nutrition: it is true that xviiith and nineteenth ° For centuries, I did not believe that the consumption of meat was absolutely necessary for the man, because monks He abstained all the time and the most peasants almost never knew. The caste of Brahmins, vegetarian for millennia, did not die either, and remember Voltaire" .

Currently, some industrially produced meats contain traces of industrial products ingested by animals or inoculated with them during their lifetime (growth hormones (not in Europe), antibiotics, contraceptives and pesticides). It should be noted that the use of hormones (growth or otherwise), common in the United States, is prohibited in Canada and France.

The meat of animals raised with hormones (especially cows and fattened pigs) contains higher water content and provides lower nutritional value than animals living freely in their natural environment. This reality brings a number of people to become vegetarians.

False news opposite vegetarianism

According to Marie-Claude Marsolier-Kergoat, biologist and researcher in the National Museum of Natural History in Paris, "We know that livestock is a waste of the planet's resources, that the consumption of animal products contributes to the increase in chronic diseases and that we treat animals raised, hunted or fished with cruelty. "false information" (" false news ") the opposition of vegetarians would be transmitted consistently by the majority of Western public opinion, as well as by the media (such as Fox News) and the popular scientific press.

"The extension in time and in all the components of our societies of these false news , which seek to disqualify vegetarianism both physiologically and ethically, may surprise. Where does this general appetite for women come from? anti-vegetarian rhetoric despite their irrational nature? It is likely that most people feel an incoherence between their claims to "respect" or even "to love" animals or nature and their eating behavior.The tension induced by this type of Cognitive dissonance can be mitigated by several strategies, including denial of facts and denigration of the people who expose them.

Literature and cinema

In From Rene Barjavel novel The night of time , the heroine Elea is horrified to learn that humans today "eat the beast". In fact, the people to which it belongs, with the exception of the marginal or asocial life outside the system, do not consume animals but synthetic foods produced by a "dining machine" which miraculously works according to the equation of Zoran (it is for Therefore, beyond vegetarianism, do not consume natural foods, but only artificial foods.

In the legacy cycle , the hero becomes a vegetarian during his training as Dragon Elf, themselves lacto-ovo-vegetarians. He will end up eating meatlessly when, in the middle of the desert, he will have no choice but to sacrifice the life of two lizards to survive the crossing.

In the saga of the Emerald Knights and his suite, the heirs of the elves and fairies of Enkidiev, even those who are knights, are vegetarians. The gentleman Kevin, after getting rid of the magician Asbeth who had mutated him (who had woken up with the death of the magician) and who had made him exclusively crud-carnivorous and blind under a bright light , becomes a vegetarian at the insistent request of his wife Maïwen (a fairy) and his children, and eventually get used to this new regime.

In La Belle Verte , from and with Coline Serreau , Mila and all her community are vegetarians.

In The Simpsons , Lisa, daughter of Homer and Marge, becomes a vegetarian.

Mythes of the Vegetarianism

Bill and Tania sat in front of me in my office in a dark mood: they had just lost their first baby in the second month of pregnancy. Tania was very upset: "Why did that happen to me, why did I make my baby stumble?" The young couple came to see me mainly because of Tania's repeated respiratory infections but she also wanted some tips on how to avoid the sadness of another lost pregnancy.

While I was wondering about Tania's diet, I quickly understood the cause of her infections, as well as her miscarriage: she was not essentially fat in her diet and she was also mostly vegetarian. Due to the abundant media rhetoric about the perceived risks of consuming animal products, contrary to the alleged benefits of the vegetarian lifestyle for health, Tania deliberately removed foods such as cream, butter, meat and fish. Although he loved the liver, he avoided it because of concerns about "toxins".

Tania and Bill left with a bottle of vitamin A, with other supplements and a recipe in foods that contained large amounts of animal fat and meat. Shortly before I left my office, Tania looked at me and said sadly: "I do not know what to believe sometimes." Wherever I look, we recommend all these low-fat vegetarians, I followed them and I saw what happened. " I assured her that if she and her husband changed their diet and given enough time to weaken the uterus to heal, they would be happy parents in due course. In November 2000, Bill and Tania gave birth to their first child, a girl.

The evolution of a myth

Along with unjustified and unscientific fears about saturated fat and cholesterol in recent decades, it has become clear that vegetarianism is a healthier nutritional choice for man. It seems that every health expert and state health service urges people to consume fewer animal products and consume more vegetables, seeds, fruits and legumes. These prompts are supplemented by confirmations and studies supposedly demonstrating that vegetarianism is healthier for the people and that meat consumption is associated with illness and death. However, many authorities questioned these elements, but their objections were largely ignored.

As we shall see, many vegetarian allegations can not be justified and some are simply false and dangerous. Vegetarian diets have benefits for certain health conditions, and some people work better with less fat and protein, but as a professional who has been involved with several former vegetarians and vegans, I know the dangerous effects of a diet that does not have healthy animals products. I hope that all readers will soon examine their position on vegetarianism after reading this Chapter.

CONSUMPTION OF MEAT CONTRIBUTES TO HUNGER AND EXHAUSTS THE NATURAL RESOURCES OF THE EARTH.

Some vegetarians have argued that animals require grassland that can be used to grow grain to feed hungry people in Third World countries. It is also argued that animal feed contributes to hunger in the world because the animals eat food that could be used to feed people. The solution to hunger in the world is therefore to become a vegetarian. These arguments are absurd and simple.

The first argument ignores the fact that about two-thirds of the land on our planet is not suitable for agriculture. These are mainly open areas, deserts and mountainous areas which provide feed for grazing livestock and these lands are currently used wisely.

The second argument is also wrong because it ignores the vital contribution of farm animals to the well-being of humanity. It is also misleading to believe that food produced for animal feed could be diverted to human nutrition:
"Animals have always contributed to the well-being of human societies by providing food, shelters, fuels, fertilizers and other products and services." They are a renewable resource and use another renewable resource, plant, to produce these products and services. In addition, manure produced by livestock contributes to soil fertility and therefore helps plants. In some developing countries, manure can not be used as a fertilizer but is dried as a fuel source.

"Many people think that because the world's population grows faster than food supplies, we are less able to buy food of animal origin because the diet of plant products is inefficient use of potential human food. It is true that it is more effective for people to they consume plant products directly instead of allowing animals to be converted into human food, a pound or less of human food per kilogram of plants consumed, Effectiveness applies only to plants and plant products that man can use, since more than two-thirds of the animal feed consists of substances that are undesirable or totally unfit for human consumption Non-edible plant material for human consumption, not they just do not compete with the animals but they also contribute significantly to improving both the quantity and quality of nutrition of human societies. "

In addition, at the moment, the food produced in the world is more than enough to feed all the inhabitants of the planet. The problem is the widespread poverty that prevents hungry poor people from providing the means themselves. In a comprehensive report, the Population Reporting Office attributed the problem of world hunger to poverty rather than meat consumption . Nor does it consider massive vegetarianism a hunger solution in the world.

But what would happen if livestock farming was abandoned in favor of mass cultivation, which came from the humanity that turned to vegetarianism?

"If a large number of people switch to vegetarianism, if the demand for meat in the United States and Europe is reduced, cereal supply will increase significantly, but the purchasing power of poor [hungry] Asia will not change at all.

"The result would be very predictable - there will be a huge outflow of agriculture. While the total quantity of grain produced could feed 10 billion people, the total amount of grain produced in the world will probably fall to around 7 or 8 billion. The tendency of farmers to sell their land to developers and others will accelerate quickly.

In other words, there would be less food to eat in the world. In addition, cereal and legume monoculture, which would happen if the breeding was abandoned and the world relies solely on plant foods, would quickly hit the soil and would require intensive use of artificial fertilizers, including one tonne requiring the production of ten tons of crude oil).

As far as the impact on our environment is concerned, a closer look reveals the significant damage that could be caused by exclusive and mass cultivation. The British producer of organic dairy products and researcher Mark Purdey unambiguously stresses that "if farm systems of farming were damaged in the soil, agrochemical use, soil erosion, health problems would deteriorate" .

Neanderthin's author, Ray Audette, shares this opinion:

"Since antiquity, the most devastating factor of environmental degradation has been monoculture: the production of wheat in the ancient sameria has transformed the former fertile plains into alluvial plains that remain sterile 5000 years later." In addition to exhaustion of soil and monoculture, agriculture it is also detrimental to the environment by altering the delicate balance of natural ecosystems. For example, world rice production in 1993 caused 155 million malaria cases a fertile ground for the multiplication of mosquitoes in rice fields, rice fields have caused 500 million cases of influenza in the same year ".

There is no doubt, however, that methods of commercial production, either plant or animal, are harmful to the environment. In view of the intensive use of agrochemicals, pesticides, artificial fertilizers, hormones, steroids and antibiotics in modern agriculture, a better way of incorporating agriculture. One possible solution could be the return to "mixed agriculture", which is described below:

The educated consumer and the illuminated farmer together can contribute to the return of the mixed farm, where the cultivation of fruits, vegetables and seeds is combined with livestock and poultry effectively, economically and For example, wild hens in the garden areas eat parasites by providing high quality eggs, pastures in orchards eliminate the need for herbicides and cows grazing in the forests and Other marginal areas provide rich and clean milk, making these so economically viable. Land is not the animal culture that leads to hunger and hunger, but to bad agricultural practices and monopoly distribution systems.

The "mixed farm" is also healthier for the soil, which will yield more crops if it manages according to traditional instructions. Mark Purdey made it clear that a mixed farm would provide up to five crops a year, while a "monoculture" would produce only one or two crops.

Which farm produces more food for the peoples of the world? Purdey sums up the ecological horror of "battery" and suggests future solutions by saying:

Our agricultural activities could very much prohibit farmers who are commercially charged from managing intensive livestock units, accumulators and bureaucracy with all waste, hardness, hardness, anti-sludge systems, drug-induced immunotoxicity / chemicals resulting in BSE and Salmonella, grubbing up the rainforest, etc. Our future leadership must harm the right and happy mixed medium

Farming, reviving the old traditional extended system as a basic framework, then boosting productivity to respond to today's demands by incorporating a more modern application of biological sciences into farming systems.

It does not appear that reproduction, when properly applied, is harmful to the environment. Nor does it seem that global vegetarianism or the exclusive use of agriculture to provide the world with food is a feasible or ecologically good idea.

Vitamin B12 can be obtained from plant sources

Of all myths, it is probably the most dangerous. While lactose and lactose vegetarians have sources of vitamin B12 in their diet (dairy products and eggs), vegans (vegetarians in general) do not. Vegans that do not supplement their vitamin B12 diet will eventually develop anemia (a life-threatening illness) as well as serious damage to the nervous and digestive system. most, if not all, vegans have a change in vitamin B12 metabolism, and each study of vegan groups has shown low levels of vitamin B12 in most individuals. Several studies have been conducted on the deficiencies of B12 vitamins in vegan children, often with disastrous consequences. In addition, the vegetarian and vegetarian literature suggests that B12 is present in some seaweed, tempeh (a soy fermented product) and brewer's yeast. Everything is false because vitamin B12 is found only in food of animal origin. Beers and nutritional doughs do not contain natural vitamin B12. They are always enriched by an external source.

There is no real vitamin B12 in plant sources, but B12 analogues - are similar to actual vitamin B12, but they are not exactly the same and therefore are not bioavailable . It should be noted here that these B12 analogues may interfere with the absorption of the actual vitamin B12 in the body due to the competitive absorption, which puts vegetarians and vegetarians who consume a lot of soy, seaweed and yeast.

Some vegetarian principles claim that vitamin B12 is produced by some fermenting bacteria in the lower intestines. This can be true, but in a form that can not be used by the body. Vitamin B12 requires an inherent stomach agent for good absorption in the ileum. Since the bacterial product has no intrinsic factor, it can not be absorbed.

It is true that Hindus living in certain areas of India do not suffer from vitamin B12 deficiency. This has led some to the conclusion that herbal foods provide this vitamin. However, this conclusion is misleading because many plants, wings, eggs, larvae and / or remains remain in the plant food they consume due to the non-use of pesticides and cleaning methods. ineffective. This is the way these people take vitamin B12. This claim is confirmed by the fact that when the Hindu Hindu Hindu immigrated back to England, megaloblastic anemia survived within a few years. In England, food is cleaner and insect residues are completely eliminated by plants.

The only reliable and absorbable sources of vitamin B12 are animal products, especially offal and eggs. Although they are in quantities smaller than meat and eggs, dairy products contain vitamin B12. Therefore, Vegans should consider adding dairy products to their diet. If dairy products are not tolerated, eggs, preferably from free-range hens, are a virtual necessity.

The fact that vitamin B12 can only be taken from food of animal origin is one of the strongest arguments against veganism as a "natural" medium of human consumption. Today, vegans can avoid anemia by taking vitamin supplements or fortified foods. If these same people had lived a few decades ago when these products were not available, they would be dead.

Our needs for Vitamin D can be covered by sunlight

Although it is not really a vegetarian myth, it is widely accepted that one can satisfy the needs of a vitamin D by simply exposing his skin to the sunlight for 15-20 minutes several times a week. Vitamin D deficiencies in vegetarians and vegans are still important because this nutritional substance, in a complex form, is found only in animal fats that do not consume vegans and that moderate vegetarians do not consume. they consume only in limited quantities due to their meat-free diet.

It is true that a limited number of herbal foods such as alfalfa, sunflower seeds and avocados contain the plant form of vitamin D (ergocalciferol or vitamin D2). Although D2 can be used to prevent and treat vitamin D deficiency, rickets in humans can be wondered if this form is as effective as vitamin D3 (cholecalciferol) derived from the animal. Some studies have shown that D2 is not used as D3 in animals and clinicians have reported disappointing effects using vitamin D2 to treat vitamin D-related conditions .

Although vitamin D can be created by our body through the action of sun on our skin, it is very difficult to achieve an optimal amount of vitamin D with a brief invasion of the sun. Ultraviolet rays A, B and C are derived from sunlight. Only form "B" is able to catalyze the conversion of cholesterol to vitamin D in our body , and UV-B rays are present only. At certain times of the day, at certain latitudes and at certain times of the year. In addition, depending on the color of the skin, taking 200 to 400 IU of vitamin D from the sun may take up to two hours of full sunlight . Therefore, a vegan with dark skin will not be able to get the optimal intake of vitamin D with sunbathing for 20 minutes several times a week, even if this sunshine occurs during the times of the day and the sun. year when UV-B radiation is available. .

The current RDA for vitamin D is 400 IU, but the basic research of Dr. Weston Price for adult healthy adult nutrition showed that daily vitamin D (feed) was about 10 times higher, 4,000 IU. As a result, Price has put a lot of emphasis on vitamin D in its diet. Without vitamin D, for example, it is impossible to use minerals such as calcium, phosphorus and magnesium. Recent research confirmed the highest recommendations of Dr. Price for vitamin D in adults.

Since many vegetarians and vegans have documented rickets and / or low levels of vitamin D , animal fats either are inadequate or inadequate in vegetarian diets (as well as those in the general western try to systematically reduce their consumption) . animal fats) because sunlight is a source of vitamin D only at certain times and at certain latitudes and given that the current dietary recommendations for vitamin D are too low, we stress the need for reliable sources and abundant nutrients in our daily our life. regimes. Good sources include cod liver oil, pork lard that has been exposed from the sun, shrimp, wild salmon, sardines, butter, fatty dairy products and well-fed chicken eggs.

The needs of vitamin a in the body can be derived from plant foods.

True vitamin A or retinol and its related esters are found only in animal fats and organs such as the liver . Plants contain β-carotene, a substance that the body can convert to vitamin A if there are certain conditions .

Beta-carotene, however, is not vitamin A. It is typical for vegetarians and vegetarians (like most popular nutritionists) to say that plant foods such as carrots and spinach contain vitamin A and that beta-carotene is so good as vitamin. These things are not true, although β-carotene is an important nutrient for humans.

The conversion of carotene to vitamin A in the intestines can only take place in the presence of bile salts. This means that fat should be consumed with carotenes to stimulate bile secretion. In addition, infants and individuals with hypothyroidism, gall bladder problems or diabetes (a large proportion of the total population) can not convert or do little. Finally, transforming the body into carotene in vitamin A is not very effective: it takes about 6 carotene units to become a vitamin A unit. This means that a sweet potato (containing about 25,000 beta-carotene units) converts it to about 4,000 units vitamin A (assuming you eat it with fat, you are not a diabetic, you are not an infant and you have no thyroid problem) or gall bladder).

Trust in plant sources for vitamin A is not a good idea. This is another reason to include feed and fats in our diet. Butters and fatty dairy products, especially those from grazing, are good sources of vitamin A, cod liver oil. Vitamin A is essential in our diet because it allows the body to use proteins and minerals, ensures good vision, strengthens the immune system, allows reproduction and fights infections.

As with Vitamin D, Dr. Price found that diets of healthy primitive people provided significant amounts of vitamin A, highlighting once again the great need of people to maintain this nutrient for optimal health now and for generations to come.

Meat consumption causes osteoporosis, kidney disease, heart disease and cancer.

Vegans and vegetarians often try to prevent people from avoiding animal feeds and fats by claiming that vegetarian diets offer protection against certain chronic diseases such as those listed above. Such statements, however, are difficult to reconcile with historical and anthropological facts. All of the diseases mentioned are mainly cases of the 20th century, but people have been eating meat and animal fat for thousands of years. Moreover, as the Price survey showed, many indigenous populations around the world (Innuit, Maasai, Switzerland, etc.) had a traditional diet that was very rich in animal products but did not suffer. the aforementioned diseases. The independent studies by Dr. George Mann of Maasai, conducted many years after Dr. Price, confirmed that Maasai, although eating almost exclusively meat, nevertheless had heart disease or other illnesses. chronic, minor or even zero conditions.

This proves that other factors than feed are at the root of these diseases.

Several studies have shown that meat consumption is the cause of various diseases, but such studies, which are honestly evaluated, show nothing of the sort that is presented in the following discussion.

Osteoporosis

The research of Dr. Herta Spencer on protein intake and bone loss clearly showed that protein intake in the form of real meat had no impact on bone density. Studies believed to indicate that excessive protein consumption resulted in increased bone loss was not performed with real meat, but with fractionated protein powders and isolated amino acids. Recent studies have also shown that increased consumption of animal proteins contributes to increasing bone density in both men and women. However, recent studies on diet of vegetarians and vegetarians have shown that they predispose women to osteoporosis.

Hospital Disease

Although limited protein diets are useful for people with renal insufficiency, there is no indication that meat is the cause. Vegetarians also generally claim that animal proteins cause too much acidic conditions in the blood, resulting in rinsing of bone calcium and, therefore, a higher tendency to form kidney stones. This theory is false, however, theoretically, sulfur and phosphorus in meat can form acid when placed in water, but that does not mean that it is happening in the body. In fact, the meat contains whole proteins and vitamin D (if we eat skin and fats), which help maintain the balance of blood pH. In addition, if you consume a diet containing enough magnesium and vitamin B6 and restrict refined sugars, you should not worry about kidney stones, whether eating or not. Feed like beef, pork, fish and lamb are good sources of magnesium and vitamin B6, as shown in any table of nutrients and nutrients.

Heart deseases

The belief that animal protein contributes to heart disease is a popular idea that has no foundation in the science of nutrition. In addition to questionable studies, there is little evidence to support the idea that eating meat causes heart disease. For example, the French have one of the highest per capita consumption of meat but have low rates of heart disease. In Greece, meat consumption is above average, but heart disease rates are also low. Finally, in Spain, the increase in meat consumption (associated with reduced sugar and high carbohydrate intake) has led to a reduction in heart disease.

Cancer

The belief that meat, especially red meat, contributes to cancer is, like heart disease, a popular idea that is not supported by the facts. While it is true that some studies have shown a relationship between eating meat and certain types of cancer, it is important to look carefully at these studies to determine the type of meat under discussion. as well as the manufacturing methods used. Since we have only one word for "meat" in English, it is often difficult to know which "meat" is being discussed in a study unless the authors of the study specifically say it.

The study that started the theory of meat = cancer was conducted by Dr. Ernst Wynder in the 1970s . Wynder claimed that there was a direct causal link between the consumption of animal fat and the incidence of colorectal cancer. In fact, its data on "animal fats" were indeed related to vegetable fats. In other words, cancer theory = cancer is based on a false study.

If we look closely at the research, we will quickly see that it is processed meat, such as cold cuts and sausages that are generally involved in the causality of cancer and not in the meat itself. In addition, cooking methods appear to play a role in meat cancer . In other words, it is the chemicals added to the meat and the chosen cooking method and not the meat itself.

In the end, although there is sometimes a relationship between meat and cancer, the mechanism itself has escaped. This means that it is likely that factors other than meat play a role in some cases of cancer. Remember: studies of traditional people eating meat show that they have a very small number of cancers. This indicates that other factors begin to play when cancer occurs in a modern person who eats meat. It is not scientifically correct to distinguish a food factor by blaming ourselves while ignoring other potential candidates.

It should be noted here that Seventh-day Adventists are often studied in population analyzes for show that vegetarian diet is healthier and has a lower risk of cancer next paragraph in this section). If it is true that most members of this Christian confession do not eat meat, smoke or drink alcohol, coffee or tea, which can lead to cancer.

It's just a matter of looking at how it works to make it easier for you to get started. Although their church requires moderation, Mormons are not left out of the meat. Commit you to Adventists, Mormons also eagerly give you tobacco, alcohol and coffee. As well as mangeing of the meat, the South Mormons from Utah found that they were presenting a taux of cancer in general 22% plus feasible and mortality from cancer of the lower limb of 34% to moyenne américaine.

Similar results can be obtained to show that the consumption of meat and animal fat is not correlated with cancer. Obviously, other factors are at work.

It is generally argued that vegetarians have a lower cancer rate than carnivores, but a 1994 study of vegetarian vegetarian Adventists in California showed that although they had lower rates for some cancers (by example, breast and lung), they were higher. several others (Hodgkin's disease, malignant melanoma, brain, skin, uterus, prostate, endometrium, cervical and ovarian), some quite significantly. In this study, the authors admitted that:

"Meat consumption, however, was not associated with a higher [cancer] risk."

And that,

"No significant association between breast cancer and high consumption of animal fats or animal products in general was noted."

In addition, it is generally claimed that a diet rich in plant foods, such as whole grains and legumes, will reduce the risk of cancer, but research from the last century shows that carbohydrate diets are the main instigators of cancer. cancer, not diets. on low-processed animal foods.

The mainstream health media and vegetarian media have done such an effective job of "smearing the beef," that most people think that meat, especially red meat, is not healthy. In fact, however, animal-based foods such as beef and lamb are excellent sources of a variety of nutrients, as shown in any table of foods/ nutrients. Nutrients such as vitamins A, D, several B complex compounds, essential fatty acids (in small amounts), magnesium, zinc, phosphorus, potassium, iron, taurine and selenium are abundant in the body. beef, lamb, pork, fish and shellfish. and poultry. Nutritional factors such as coenzyme Q10, carnitine and alpha-lipoic acid are also present. Some of these nutrients are found only in foods of animal origin - the plants do not provide them.

Saturated fats and dietary cholesterol cause heart disease, atherosclerosis and / or cancer, and diets low in fat and cholesterol are healthier for humans.

Nor is it a specific vegetarian myth. Nevertheless, people are often invited to follow a vegetarian or vegan diet, because it is thought that these diets offer protection against heart disease and cancer because they are less rich or less rich in foods and fats.

Although saturated fats and dietary cholesterol are generally thought to "clog the arteries" and cause heart disease, such ideas have been proven wrong by scientists such as Linus Pauling, Russell Smith, George Mann, John Yudkin, Abram Hoffer, Enig Mary, Uffe Ravnskov and other eminent researchers.

On the contrary, studies have shown that arterial plaque is mainly composed of unsaturated fatty acids, in particular polyunsaturated fatty acids, and not saturated fatty acids of animals, palm or coconut.

Researchers such as Enig, Mann, and Fred Kummerow have demonstrated that trans fatty acids, as factors responsible for accelerated atherosclerosis, coronary heart disease, cancer, and other conditions. Trans fatty acids are found in modern foods such as margarine, vegetable shortening and foods made with. Enig and his colleagues have also shown that excessive intake of omega- 6 polyunsaturated fatty acids from refined vegetable oils is also a major contributor to cancer and heart disease, not animal fats.

A recent study of thousands of Swedes corroborated Enig's findings and data and showed no correlation between saturated fat intake and increased risk of breast cancer. However, the study, like Enig's work, showed a close link between vegetable oil consumption and higher rates of breast cancer.

The main population studies that are supposed to prove the theory that animal fats and cholesterol cause heart disease do not disappear more closely. The Framingham Heart Study is often cited as evidence that dietary cholesterol and saturated fat intake causes heart disease and poor health. Involving about 6,000 people, the study compared two groups over several years at five-year intervals. One group consumed little cholesterol and saturated fat, while the other consumed large amounts. Surprisingly, Dr. William Castelli, director of the study, said:

In Framingham, Massachusetts, the more we eat saturated fat, the more we eat cholesterol, the more we eat calories, the lower the serum cholesterol level of the person ... we found that the people who ate the most cholesterol, ate the most saturated fats, [and] ate the most calories, weighed the least, and were the most physically active.

Framingham data showed that subjects with higher cholesterol and higher weight had a slightly higher risk of coronary heart disease.However, weight gain and serum cholesterol levels were inversely correlated with intake of dietary lipids and cholesterol. In other words, there was no correlation.

In the same vein, the American Multiple Risk Factor Study, sponsored by the National Heart and Lung Institute, compared mortality rates and dietary habits of more than 12,000 men. Those who ate less saturated fat and cholesterol had a slightly reduced heart rate, but a much higher overall mortality rate than the other men in the study.

Diets low in fat and cholesterol are therefore not healthier for people. Studies have repeatedly shown that such diets are associated with depression, cancer, psychological problems, fatigue, violence and suicide.

Women with low serum cholesterol have shorter lives than women with higher rates. Similar things have been found among men.
Children on a low-fat and / or vegan diet may suffer from growth problems, growth failure and learning disabilities. Despite this, sources from Dr. Benjamin Spock of the American Heart Association recommend low fat diets for children! We can only deplore the fate of these unfortunate young people who will be raised by ignorant parents supported by such genocidal disinformation.

Saturated fats have many health benefits, depending on the fat in question. Coconut oil, for example, is rich in lauric acid, antifungal and potent antimicrobial substance. Coconut also contains appreciable amounts of caprylic acid, also an effective antifungal.

Cow butter is rich in trace elements, especially selenium, and all the fat-soluble vitamins and beneficial fatty acids that protect against cancer and fungal infections.

In fact, the body needs saturated fats to properly use essential fatty acids. Saturated fats also lower blood levels of lipoprotein damaging the arteries; are necessary for a good use of calcium in bones; stimulate the immune system; are the preferred foods of the heart and other vital organs ; and, with cholesterol, adds structural stability to the cell and intestinal wall.

They are excellent for cooking because they are chemically stable and do not decompose on heat, unlike polyunsaturated vegetable oils. To omit them from one's diet is therefore ill-advised.

With regard to atherosclerosis, it is always claimed that vegetarians have much lower rates of this disease than meat eaters. However, the International Atherosclerosis Project of 1968, which examined more than 20,000 corpses in several countries, concluded that vegetarians had as much atherosclerosis as meat eaters. Other population studies have revealed similar data.

Indeed, atherosclerosis is largely unrelated to diet; it is a consequence of aging. There are factors that can accelerate the atherosclerotic process, such as excessive damage to the arteries by free radicals due to antioxidant depletion (caused by smoking, poor diet, excess of polyunsaturated fatty acids in the diet, various nutritional deficiencies, medications, etc.), but this must be distinguished from the fatty streaks and hardening of the arteries that occur in all peoples over time.

It also does not seem that vegetarian diets protect against heart disease. A 1970 vegan study showed that mortality rates for heart disease were higher among women than among non-vegan women.

A recent study has shown that although they are vegetarians, Indians have very high rates of coronary heart disease . Diets high in carbohydrates and low in fat (which are vegetarian diets) can also increase the risk of heart disease, diabetes and cancer because of their hyperinsulemic effects on the body.

Recent studies have also shown that vegetarians have higher blood levels of homocysteine.

Homocysteine is a known cause of heart disease. Finally, Studies that conclude that vegetarians have a lower risk of heart disease generally rely on dummy markers of reduced saturated fat intake, lower serum cholesterol levels, and HDL / LDL ratios. Since vegetarians tend to eat less saturated fats and generally have lower serum cholesterol levels, it is concluded that their risk of heart disease is lower. Once it is realized that these measures are not accurate predictors of susceptibility to heart disease, the supposed protection of vegetarianism disappears.

It must always be remembered that a number of factors influence the development of heart disease or cancer in a person. Instead of focusing on the dummy problems of saturated fat, dietary cholesterol and meat consumption, people should pay more attention to other more likely factors.

These would be trans fatty acids, excessive intake of polyunsaturated fats, excessive sugar intake, excessive carbohydrate intake, smoking, certain vitamin and mineral deficiencies, and obesity. These things were all missing from the traditional healthy people studied by Dr. Price.

Vegetarians live longer and have more energy and stamina than meat eaters.

A vegetarian guide published in Britain stated that:

"You and your children do not need to eat meat to stay healthy, in fact, vegetarians say they are among the healthiest people and can expect to live nine years longer than the meat. eaters (this is often because cardiac and circulatory diseases are rarer). According to a survey conducted by the Food Research Association in January 1990, almost half of the British population is currently trying to avoid meat. "

Commenting on this extended life claim, author Craig Fitzroy astutely points out that:

"The nine-year advantage" is anecdotal evidence of vegetarianism, often repeated but still without source. But anyone who believes that by snubbing his mother's Sunday roast, he will add a decade to his years on the planet, is almost certainly seduced a little wishful thinking. "

And that's what most claims for increased longevity for vegetarians are: anecdotal. There is no evidence that a healthy vegetarian diet, compared to a balanced, omnivorous diet, prolongs life. In addition, people who choose a vegetarian lifestyle generally choose not to smoke, but rather to exercise, to lead a healthier life. These factors also affect longevity.

In the scientific literature, there are surprisingly few studies on vegetarian longevity. Russell Smith, PhD, in his review of heart disease, showed that when animal consumption increased in some study groups, death rates actually decreased! Such results have not been obtained in vegetarian subjects. For example, in a study published by Burr and Sweetnam in 1982, the analysis of mortality data revealed that, although the rate of heart disease was slightly (0.11%) lower than that of non-vegetarians, the rate All-cause mortality was much higher among vegetarians. for vegetarians.

Despite claims that studies have shown that meat consumption increases the risk of heart disease and shortens lives, the authors of these studies actually found the opposite. For example, in a 1984 analysis of a 1978 study of Seventh-day Adventist vegetarians, HA Kahn concluded:

"Although our findings add some substantial facts to the issue of diet-related diseases, we recognize how far they are from establishing, for example, that men who eat meat frequently or women who rarely eat of salad thus shorten their life. "

DA Snowden reached a similar conclusion . Despite these surprising admissions, the studies nevertheless concluded exactly the opposite and urged people to reduce animal foods from their diet.

In addition, these two studies eliminated some dietary data that clearly did not show any relationship between eggs, cheese, whole milk, and meat-related fat (all foods high in cholesterol and fat) and heart disease. . Dr. Smith commented,

"In fact, the Kahn [and Snowden] study is another example of negative results massaged and misinterpreted to corroborate the politically correct claims that vegetarians are living longer."

Meat eating people are generally said to be short-lived, but Australian Aborigines, who traditionally eat a diet rich in animal products, are known for their longevity (at least before European colonization). In Aboriginal society, there is a special caste of elderly people. Obviously, if there were no seniors, no such group would have existed. In his book Nutrition and Physical Degeneration, Dr. Price has many photographs of seniors peoples of the world. Explorers such as Vilhjalmur Stefansson have reported a great longevity among the Innuit (again, before colonization).

Likewise, Russians in the Caucasus Mountains live for a very long time on a diet consisting of fatty pork and whole milk products. Hunzas, also known for their robust health and longevity, consume substantial portions of goat's milk that has a higher saturated fat content than cow's milk.

By contrast, the largely vegetarian Hindus of southern India have the shortest life span in the world, partly because of a lack of food, but also because of a clear lack of animal protein in their diet.

The comments of H. Leon Abrams are instructive here:

"Vegetarians often argue that a diet consisting of meat and animal fat leads to a death. The anthropological data of primitive societies do not support such claims. "

In terms of endurance and energy levels, Dr. Price traveled the world in the 1920s and 1930s to study the diet of aboriginals. Without exception, he found a strong correlation between diets rich in animal fats, robust health and athletic abilities. Special dishes for Swiss athletes, for example, included bowls of fresh and raw cream. In Africa, Dr. Price found that groups whose diet was rich in fatty meat and fish, and offal such as liver, consistently won prizes in sports competitions, and that meat-eating tribes still dominated. tribes whose diet was largely vegetarian.

In the field of sports nutrition, it is common to recommend that "athletes" increase their level of endurance. However, recent studies in New York and South Africa show that the opposite is true: "carbohydrate-loaded" athletes had significantly less stamina than those "fat-laden" before sporting events.

The diet of the "caveman" was low in fat and / or vegetarian. Humans have evolved as vegetarians.

Our ancestors of the Paleolithic were hunter-gatherers and three schools of thought developed to define their diet. One group advocates for a high-fat, animal-based diet supplemented with seasonal fruits, berries, nuts, root vegetables and wild herbs. The second asserts that primitive peoples consumed an assortment of lean meats and large quantities of plant foods. The third affirms that our human ancestors evolved as vegetarians.

Drs. Loren Cordain and Boyd Eaton, Ph.D., voraciously advocated "lean" diets in a number of popular and professional publications.

Cordain and Eaton believe in the lipid hypothesis of heart disease - the belief (refuted in myth number six above) that saturated fat and dietary cholesterol contribute to heart disease. Because of this and the fact that Paleolithic peoples or their modern equivalents suffer / do not suffer from heart disease, Cordain and Eaton subscribe to the theory that Paleolithic peoples consume most of their fat calories from monounsaturated and polyunsaturated sources. and unsaturated fats. Believing that saturated fats are dangerous for our arteries, Cordain and Eaton remain in step with the current nutritional thinking of the institutions and encourage modern peoples to adopt a diet comparable to that of our ancestors. They believe that this diet was rich in lean meats and a variety of vegetables, but low in saturated fats. The evidence they produce to support this theory is, however, very selective and misleading.

Saturated fats do not cause heart disease, as shown above, and our Paleolithic ancestors ate a lot of saturated fats from different animal sources. And our Paleolithic ancestors ate some saturated fat from various animal sources. and our Paleolithic ancestors ate some saturated fat from various animal sources.

From authoritative sources, we learn that prehistoric humans from the North American continent have eaten animals such as mammoth, camel, sloth, bison, mountain sheep, American antelope, beaver, moose, mule deer and llama. "Mammoths, sloths, mountain sheep, bison and beavers are modern fat animals because they have a thick layer of subcutaneous fat, as do the many species of bears and wild pigs whose remains have been found at Paleolithic sites around the world. "

The analysis of many types of game fat such as antelope, bison, caribou, dog, elk, moose, seal and mountain sheep shows that they are rich in saturated and monounsaturated fatty acids, but relatively low in polyesters.

In addition, although buffaloes and game may have lean, non-marbled muscle flesh, it is wrong to assume that only these parts were consumed by hunter-gatherer groups such as Native Americans who often hunted animals selectively. for their fatty and fatty organs. the next section will show.

Anthropologists / explorers such as Vilhjalmur Stefansson have reported that the Innu and Indian tribes of North America would be worried when their caribou catches were too thin: they knew that the disease would follow if they did not consume enough. In other words, these primitive people did not like to eat lean meat.

Indians in the Canadian North also deliberately hunted older caribou and elk, as these animals carried a 50-pound fat plate that the Indians ate with taste. This "dorsal fat" is highly saturated. Native Americans would also refrain from hunting bison in the spring (when the fat reserves of these animals were low, due to lack of food in winter), preferring to hunt, kill and consume them in the fall when were fattened.

The explorer Samuel Hearne, writing in 1768, described how the Native American tribes with whom he came in contact selectively hunted caribou only for fat parties:

"On July 22, we met several foreigners, whom we joined in pursuit of the caribou, who were so numerous at the time that we received a sufficient number of people every day for our support, and that we killed all too often just several languages, marrow and fat. "

Although Cordain and Eaton are certainly right in saying that our ancestors ate meat, their assertions about fat consumption, as well as the type of fat consumed, are simply inaccurate.

While various vegetarian and vegan authorities like to think that we have evolved as a species on a vegan or vegetarian diet, there is very little anthropology of nutrition to support these ideas.

For starters, in his travels, Dr. Price has never found a totally vegetarian culture. It is worth remembering that Mr. Price visited and studied several population groups that were, for all intents and purposes, the 20th century equivalents of our hunter-gatherer ancestors . Dr. Price was looking for a vegetarian culture, but he came empty. Price indicated:

"I have not yet found a primitive racial group that builds and maintains great bodies by living entirely with plant foods."

Anthropological evidence confirms this: all over the world, all societies show a preference for animal foods and fats, and our ancestors turned to large-scale farming only when they had to deal with increased demographic pressure. Abrams and other authorities have shown that it is the prehistoric man's quest for more food of animal origin that motivated his expansion on Earth and that he apparently hunted certain species up to the extinction.

Price also found that people who by necessity consumed more grains and legumes had higher rates of tooth decay than those who consumed more animal products. In his articles on vegetarianism, Abrams presents archaeological evidence to support this finding: Skulls of ancient, largely vegetarian peoples have teeth containing cavities and abscesses, as well as signs of tuberculosis and other infectious diseases. The emergence of agriculture and increased reliance on plant foods for our livelihood was clearly detrimental to our health.

Finally, it is simply impossible for our prehistoric ancestors to be vegetarians because they would not have been able to get enough calories or nutrients to survive with the available plant foods. The reason is that humans could not cook or control the fire at the time, and the vast majority of plant foods, particularly cereals and legumes, had to be cooked to make them edible. man . Most people are unaware that many of the plant foods we eat today are poisonous in their raw state.

On the basis of all this evidence, it is certain that the diets of our ancestors, the genitors of humanity, ate a very non-vegetarian diet, rich in saturated fatty acids.

Consumption of meat and saturated fats increased in the 20th century, resulting in a corresponding increase in heart disease and cancer.

Statistics do not confirm such fantasies. Butter consumption increased from 18 lb (8.665 kg) per person per year in 1900 to less than 5 lb (2.27 kg) per person per year today.

In addition, Westerners, solicited by government health agencies, reduced their consumption of eggs, cream, lard and pork. Chicken consumption has increased in recent decades, but chicken has less saturated fat than beef or pork.

In addition, an investigation of cookbooks published in the United States in the last century shows that people of ancient times ate a lot of animal foods and saturated fats. For example, in the Baptist Ladies Cook Book (Monmouth, Illinois, 1895), virtually all recipes require butter, cream or lard.

Recipes for vegetables with cream are also numerous. The Searchlight cookbook (Capper Publications, 1931) also contains similar recipes: creamy liver, creamed cucumbers, buttermilk braised hearts, and so on. British Jews, as shown by the Jewish Housewives Cookbook (London, 1846), also had diets rich in cream, butter, eggs and lamb and beef tallow. A German waffle recipe, for example, requires a dozen egg yolks and a pound of butter. An oyster pie recipe from the Baptist cookbook calls for a pint of cream and a dozen eggs, and so on.

It does not seem that people have eaten leaner diets in the last century. It is true that beef consumption has increased in recent decades, but what has also increased dramatically is the consumption of margarine and other food products containing trans-fatty acids, " "lifeless, packaged foods, processed vegetable oils. carbohydrates and refined sugar. Since we do not see chronic diseases such as cancer and heart disease in beef-eating indigenous peoples like the Maasai and Samburu, it is not possible that beef is at the root of these modern epidemics.

This, of course, points directly to other dietary factors as the most likely causes.

Soy products are suitable substitutes for meat and dairy products.

It is typical for vegetarians and vegetarians in the western world to use a variety of soy products for their protein needs. There is no doubt that the multi-billion dollar soybean industry has benefited immensely from the cholesterol and anti-meat gospel of today's nutritional thinking. While,

Not so long ago, soy was an Asian food mainly used as a condiment. Today, a variety of processed soy products are proliferating in the North American market. Although the traditionally fermented soy foods of miso, tamari, tempeh and natto are definitely healthy in measured amounts, the hyper-processed soy foods that most vegetarians consume are not.

Unfermented soybeans and foods derived from them are rich in phytic acid, an anti-nutrient that binds to minerals in the digestive tract and transports them out of the body. Vegetarians are known for their mineral deficiencies, especially zinc, and the high phytate content of cereal and legume diets is to blame.

Although several traditional food-preparation techniques, such as soaking, germination and fermentation, can significantly reduce the phytate content of cereals and legumes, such methods are not commonly known or used by indigenous peoples. modern, including vegetarians. This puts them (as well as

Soy foods are also rich in trypsin inhibitors, which hinder the digestion of proteins. Textured vegetable protein (PST), soy milk powder and soy protein, popular vegetarian milk and meat substitutes, are fully fragmented foods obtained by treating soybeans at high temperatures and washing them in different ways for extract the fat content or neutralize the power. enzyme inhibitors.

These practices completely denature the protein content of the beans, which makes them very difficult to digest. MSG, a neurotoxin, is regularly added to TVP to give it a taste identical to that of the different foods it mimics.

On a purely nutritional level, soybeans, like all legumes, are deficient in cysteine and methionine, essential amino acids containing sulfur, as well as tryptophan, another essential amino acid. In addition, soy contains no vitamins A or D, necessary for the uptake and use of bean protein by the body. It is probably for this reason that Asian cultures that consume soy often combine them with fish or fish broth (rich in fat-soluble vitamins) or other fatty foods.

Parents who feed their children with soy-based preparations should be aware of its extremely high phytoestrogen content. Some scientists have estimated that a child fed soy milk ingests the hormonal equivalent of five contraceptive pills per day.

Such consumption could have disastrous results. The soy formula also does not contain cholesterol, vital for the development of the brain and nervous system.

Although research is still ongoing, some recent studies have shown that soy phytoestrogens may be causal factors in some forms of breast cancer, congenital malformations of the penis and childhood leukemia .

Be that as it may, it has been clearly demonstrated that soy phytoestrogens, or isoflavones, impair thyroid function and cause sterility in all animal species studied so far.

It is clear that modern soy products and isolated isoflavone supplements are not healthy foods for vegetarians, vegans, or anyone else. Yet it is those who are the most consumed.

The human body is not designed for meat consumption

Some vegetarian groups claim that since humans have squeaky teeth like herbivorous animals and longer intestines than carnivorous animals, this proves that the human body is better adapted to vegetarianism.

This argument fails to note several human physiological characteristics that clearly indicate a purpose for the consumption of animal products.

First and foremost, our stomach produces hydrochloric acid, a substance that is not found in herbivores. HCL activates the protein division enzymes. In addition, the human pancreas manufactures a full range of digestive enzymes to handle a wide variety of foods, both animal and plant.

In addition, the extensive comparison of the human digestive system with the carnivorous dog and the herbivorous sheep, established by Dr. Walter Voegtlin, clearly shows that the anatomy of the carnivorous dog is closer to that of the herbivorous sheep.

Humans may have longer intestines than carnivorous animals, but they are not as long as herbivores; We also do not have multiple stomachs, like many herbivores, and we do not beg cud. Our physiology clearly indicates a mixed food or omnivore, much like our parents, the mountain gorilla and the chimpanzee, all observed eating small animals and, in some cases, other primates.

Eating animal flesh causes violent and aggressive behavior in humans.

Some vegetarian diet authorities, such as Dr. Ralph Ballantine, claim that fear and terror of an animal tried to death are somehow "transferred" into its flesh. and its organs and "becomes" a part of the person who eats it.
In addition to the fact that no scientific study supports such a theory, these thinkers would do well to recall that an irrational tendency to anger is a symptom of low vitamin B12 levels, which, as we have seen, are commonplace. in vegans. and vegetarians. In addition, during his travels, Dr. Price has always noted the extreme happiness and ungrateful nature of the people he met, who were all carnivores.

Animal products contain many harmful toxins

A recent vegetarian newsletter said:

"Most people do not realize that meat products are loaded with poisons and toxins! Meat, fish and eggs decompose and putrefy extremely fast.As soon as an animal is killed, self-destructive enzymes are released, which causes the formation of denatured substances, called ptyloamines, which cause cancer "

If meat, fish and eggs actually produce cancerous "ptyloamines", it's very strange that no one has died of cancer for millions of years. These sensational and absurd statements can not be supported by historical facts.

Hormones, nitrates and pesticides are present in livestock products (as well as in fruits, grains and vegetables), and are therefore of concern. However, these chemicals can be avoided by taking care of meat, eggs and organic dairy products, which are fed on the food and do not contain artificial and harmful toxins.

Parasites are easily avoided by taking the usual precautions in food preparations. Marinating or fermenting meat, as is customary in traditional societies, still protects against pests. During his travels, Dr. Price has always found healthy, disease-free and pest-free people, consuming raw meat and dairy products as part of their diet.

Similarly, Dr. Francis Pottenger, in his experiments on cats, showed that the healthiest and happiest cats were those on a diet consisting solely of raw foods. Cats eating cooked meats and pasteurized milk became ill and died and contained many parasites. Salmonella can be transmitted by both plant products and animals.
Vegetarians often claim that meat is harmful to our body because ammonia is released by the breakdown of its proteins. Although it is true that the digestion of the meat causes the production of ammonia, our body quickly converts this substance into harmless urea. The alleged toxicity of meat is greatly exaggerated by vegetarians.

Mad Cow Disease (BSE) is probably not caused by cows eating parts of animals with their food, which has been practiced for more than 100 years. Mark Purdey, a British farmer, has convincingly explained that cows with mad cow disease are those who have received a particular organophosphate insecticide on their backs or have suffered from soils low in magnesium, but high in aluminum.

Small cases of "mad cow disease" have also occurred in people living near cement and chemical plants and in some areas of volcanic soils.

Purdey hypothesized that organophosphate pesticides enter the fat of cows through a spraying program and are then ingested by the cows again with the animal part of the diet. Viewed in this way, it is the insecticides, via the feeder parties (and not the parties themselves or their associated "prions"), that caused this outbreak. As noted above, cows have been eating animal parts for over 100 years. It was never a problem before the introduction of these insecticides.

Purdey recently received support from Dr. Donald Brown, a British biochemist who also advocated for a non-infectious cause of BSE. Brown attributes BSE to environmental toxins, including manganese overload.

Eating meat or animal products is less "spiritual" than eating only plant-based foods.

It is often claimed that those who consume meat or animal products are less "spiritually advanced" than those who do not eat meat. Although it is not a nutritional or academic problem, those who include animal products in their diet often feel inferior. This problem therefore needs to be addressed.

Many world religions impose no restrictions on animal consumption; and neither their founders. Jews eat lamb on their holiest holiday, Passover. Muslims also celebrate Ramadan with lamb before entering their fast. Like other Jews, Jesus Christ took meat at the Last Supper (according to the canonical gospels). It is true that some forms of Buddhism impose restrictions on meat consumption, but dairy products are still allowed. Similar principles are found in Hinduism. As part of the celebration of Samhain, the Celtic pagans were slaughtering the weakest animals in the herds and tending their meat for the coming winter.

Nevertheless, it is often argued that since eating meat involves losing one's life, it is tantamount to murder. Leaving aside the religious philosophies that often permeate this issue, there seems to be a misunderstanding about the force of life and how it works. Modern peoples (vegetarians and non-vegetarians) have lost touch with what it takes to survive in our world - something Aboriginal people never lose sight of. We do not hunt or clean our meat - we buy steaks and chops at the supermarket. We do not necessarily work in the rice fields: we buy bags of brown rice; and so on and so not.

When Native Americans killed game for food, they regularly offered a prayer of thanks to the spirit of the animal that gave it life to live. In our world, life is nourished by life. Destruction is always balanced with the generation. It's a good thing: without control, the life force becomes cancerous. If the consumption of animal feed is considered in this way, it is not a murder, but a sacrifice. Modern peoples would do well to remember it.

Eating foods of animal origin is in human

Undoubtedly, some commercial livestock live in deplorable conditions where diseases and suffering are common. In countries like Korea, animals intended for consumption, such as dogs, are sometimes horribly killed, for example, beaten to death with a club. Our recommendations for the consumption of food of animal origin do not approve of such practices.

Commercial livestock farming is an unhealthy food product, whether it is meat, milk, butter, cream or eggs. Our ancestors did not eat such substandard foods, nor should we.

It is possible to raise animals humanly. This is why organic farming, preferably biodynamic, should be encouraged: it is cleaner and more efficient, and produces healthier animals and food. Each person should therefore do their utmost to purchase organically grown livestock (and plant foods). It not only supports our bodies better, because organic foods are more nutrient-dense and free of hormone and pesticide residues, but it also favors small farms and is therefore better for the economy .

Nevertheless, many people have philosophical problems to eat animal flesh, and these feelings must be respected. Dairy products and eggs, however, do not result from the death of an animal and are an excellent alternative for these people.

It must also be remembered that agriculture, which involves both the clearing of land for cultivation and the protection and maintenance of these crops, results in the death of many animals.

The belief, therefore, that "becoming a vegetarian" will somehow save the animals from death is one without any foundation.

The value of Vegetarism

As a cleansing diet, vegetarianism is sometimes a good choice. Many health problems (eg, gout) can often be improved by a temporary reduction of animal products accompanied by an increase in plant foods. But such measures should not be continuous throughout life: there are essential nutrients that should be ingested only in foods of animal origin for optimal health. In addition, there is no single diet for each person. Some vegetarians and vegans, in their zeal to get converts, are blind to this biochemical fact.

"Biochemical Individuality" is a subject that deserves to be clarified. Formulated by nutritional biochemist Roger Williams, PhD, the term refers to the fact that different people need different nutrients based on their unique genetic makeup. Ethnic and racial origin is also included in this concept. A diet that works for one may not work as well for someone else. As a practitioner, I have seen several clients on a vegetarian diet with serious health problems: obesity, candidiasis, hypothyroidism, cancer, diabetes, leaky bowel syndrome, anemia and chronic fatigue.

In addition, due to individual genetic and biochemical peculiarities, some people simply can not follow a vegetarian diet because of lectin intolerance or lack of desaturating enzymes. The lectins found in legumes, an important feature of vegetarian diets, are not tolerated by many people. Others have sensitivities to grains, especially gluten, or to grain proteins in general. Again, since cereals are a major feature of vegetarian diets, these people can not take advantage of them.

Desaturase enzyme deficiencies are generally present in persons of Inuit, Scandinavian, North European and Maritime origin. They lack the ability to convert alpha-linolenic acid to EPA and DHA, two omega-3 fatty acids that are closely involved in the functioning of the immune system and the nervous system. This is because the ancestors of these peoples drew an abundance of EPA and DHA from the large quantities of cold-water fish they ate. Over time, due to their non-use, they lost the ability to manufacture the enzymes needed to create EPA and DHA in their body. For these people, vegetarianism is simply not possible. They MUST get their EPA and DHA in food and the EPA is only found in foods of animal origin. DHA is present in some algae, but the amounts are much lower than in fish oils.

It is also clear that vegan diets are not suitable for everyone because of insufficient cholesterol production in the liver and that cholesterol is found only in foods of animal origin. It is often said that the body produces enough cholesterol and there is no reason to consume foods that contain it (animal foods). Recent research, however, has shown the opposite. Singer's work at the University of California at Berkeley has shown that cholesterol in eggs improves the memory of the elderly.

In other words, the cholesterol of these elderly people was insufficient to improve their memory, but the dietary cholesterol of the eggs was added.

Although it seems that some people do well with little or no meat and stay healthy as lacto-vegetarians or lacto-ovo-vegetarians, the reason is that these diets are healthier for these people, and not not because they are healthier in general. However, a total absence of animal products, whether meat, fish, insects, eggs, butter or dairy products, should be avoided. Although it may take years, problems will eventually arise under such diets and they will certainly appear to future generations. Dr. Price's fundamental research has demonstrated this unequivocally. The reason is a simple evolution: humanity has evolved by eating foods from animal origin and fat as part of its diet, and our body is adapted and accustomed to it. We can not change evolution in a few years.